RESEARCH PROCEDURES

in
Speech, Language, and Hearing

RESEARCH PROCEDURES

in

Speech, Language, and Hearing

William M. Shearer, Ph.D.
PROFESSOR OF COMMUNICATION DISORDERS

WILLIAMS & WILKINS
Baltimore/London

Copyright ©, 1982
Williams & Wilkins
428 East Preston Street
Baltimore, MD 21202, U.S.A.

Made in the United States of America

Library of Congress Cataloging in Publication Data

Shearer, William M.
    Research procedures in speech, language, and hearing.

    Bibliography: p.
    Includes index.
    1. Speech—Research. 2. Communicative disorders—Research. I. Title.
P95.3.S53   001.54′2   81-10389
ISBN 0-683-07724-4   AACR2

Composed and printed at the
Waverly Press, Inc.
Mt. Royal and Guilford Aves.
Baltimore, MD 21202, U.S.A.

Preface

The text is intended primarily for use in the research methodology course for graduate students in Communication Disorders and Speech and Hearing Sciences. It should serve also as a handbook for use in the advising of student research or as a convenient reference for some of the more commonly employed statistical treatments.

The general presentation assumes that the student has already had at least one course in statistics, and is now concerned mainly with the application of research principles, rather than with basic statistical theory. Since the information has been developed primarily from the experience of guiding students through their frustrations and difficulties with research papers, theses, and dissertations, the contents of these pages should have a familiar ring both to the student and to the research advisor.

The manuscript developed originally from what is now Part 3 of the text. Students needed a set of guidelines for each thesis chapter, including some tentative choices of wording to express certain concepts appropriately. As this type of advising became more repetitive, it evolved into a pamphlet which was handed to students who requested the information. Much the same circumstances arose concerning the statistical examples, and the application was expanded to meet requests related to dissertations and also to the needs of faculty colleagues.

The collection of statistical examples became the nucleus of a seminar in applied statistics, during which time the exercises were added for student use. At this point the materials assumed the role of a text, which needed broader focus and wider application, as well as discussion on the various aspects of research as a topic in itself. Thus it was that the book developed according to need, beginning as a guide to research writing, adding statistical examples, and finally addressing the subject of research and its methodology.

In contrast to most earlier texts, which have arisen from the fields of psychology, education, speech, agriculture, and biology, the format, examples, references to journals, and general discussion areas presented here are intended to give the student a clear identification with research in the field of speech, language, and hearing. Examples are drawn primarily from the *Journal of Speech and Hearing Research*, *Journal of Speech and Hearing Disorders*, and from *Language, Speech, and Hearing Services in Schools*.

My thanks to Linda Sons of the Department of Mathematics, Northern Illinois University, for the computer references used to generate some of the statistical tables, to Peter Senkowsky of the Department of Psychology for editing and checking the statistical computations, and a special note of appreciation to my wife, Marge, and to my colleagues in the Department of Communication Disorders for their support throughout the book's development and completion.

William M. Shearer, Ph.D.

Contents

Part 1
Considerations in Research Planning

Part 2
Statistical Treatment

Part 3
Research Writing

PART 1

Considerations in Research Planning

CHAPTER 1   **Introduction**

Many books have been written on the topic of research, and most start with a philosophical discussion in answer to the question, "Why do research?": Predictably, the answer turns out to be an advocation for research, because it helps the researcher to understand his field, advances the profession, and benefits society. This is, of course, true and an argument in favor of research therefore becomes much like an argument in favor of apple pie, and other things that are fundamentally good. In view of such attributes, it would seem unnecessary to promote the idea that students should become involved in research. The attributes of course do not tell the whole story; the pursuit of research must have some negative aspects. From the student's point of view, it is a major, time-consuming project that must somehow be worked into a schedule that is already overloaded. Also it is invariably an area for which the student feels poorly prepared and vulnerable to criticism and failure.

Some take the position that research is not for everyone. It has been argued that research is too open to amateurs and neophytes, and that it should be left only to those who are highly skilled and well-trained. This view was espoused in a brief, but understandably controversial editorial by Jerger, which appeared in the *Journal of Speech and Hearing Research* in 1963. In a one-page discussion entitled "Viewpoint", Jerger argued that clinicians receive extensive training to prepare them for clinical work, while research is often attempted by those who have had little or no formal training in research background or methodology. "We would like to propose that *not* everyone is competent to do research. Indeed the increasing clinical emphasis in many of our training institutions has led to progressively poorer grounding in the fundamental requisites for research." (Jerger, 1963, p. 301) Opponents of this view believe that one's potential research activity cannot be planned realistically during the basic stages of educational preparation; extensive research preparation for all would serve the needs of only a very few. In spite of academic background, the initial efforts of the beginning researcher produce manuscripts that lack the polish and sophistication that come only through experience and not necessarily through more course work.

Like most other issues, time and practical application have a way of resolving much of the concern. The student who has poor writing skills, a distaste for statistics, and little patience for detail will not join the ranks of the researchers. Similarly, the speech clinician or audiologist who has a job that assumes no research involvement does not receive the stimulation or the reward for taking on the extra chore of research and publication. For the profession at large, then, there is a self-purging influence that tends to screen out those with poor research aptitude, lack of interest, and unencouraging environment.

From a philosophical as well as practical standpoint, there is much to be said in favor of the optional Master's thesis program, as compared with those where the thesis is either required of everyone or else completely unavailable at the Master's level of study. For some students, the grudgingly completed thesis has not enhanced their Master's degree, but has served only to give their advisor an additional tutoring exercise. On the other hand, for the student with research interest and aptitude, the thesis is an invaluable early start for the research career. For some, even earlier research involvement is recommended. Depending upon the circumstances and the type of students involved, a senior thesis can be a stimulating elective to the baccalaureate curriculum, and to the aspiring young researcher.

Although the Ph.D., through the process of wholesale proliferation, has lost some of its original intent, it is still the only degree which has been designed explicitly for the purpose of training persons for a career in research. The doctoral student is, therefore, committed to the search for new knowledge when he enters the program, and a knowledge of research methodology is an essential part of the tools of his trade. In the academic environment, scientific inquiry is, so to speak, the bread of life, without which there is no means of keeping abreast of the world of rapidly changing knowledge. As students, we have all had the experience of sitting through the lectures that have been passed along from a previous time rather than developed from current information. Research at its best adds a constant newness to the field, and the cynical reference to the Ph.D. as being a "union card" applies only to those who treat it that way.

A philosophy of research which would seem both realistic and admirable was presented more than 20 years ago by Downie and Heath (1959), who said that research need not be a grim business; although tedious and demanding, it can be fun. Putting together a puzzle or solving a mystery is an invigorating and satisfying mental exercise, in which the challenge makes the goal more rewarding. Through this philosophy research may be considered as a basic human endeavor, or a natural extension of human curiosity. The authors further imply that an elitist attitude toward research may serve the purpose of maintaining a standard of quality, precision, and a healthy self-doubt in the investigator, but it becomes a tragedy to the field when anyone is frightened away from trying to solve a problem.

As any field develops, its method of synthesizing and dispensing knowledge passes through a series of fairly predictable stages. One of the earlier stages might be called the "age of authorities." At this stage, the body of knowledge is based mostly upon the observations of those who have the most experience and status in the field, typically set forth in a comprehensive text. In the speech and hearing areas, for example, the early texts were by authors such as Travis (1931), West (1937), Johnson (1946), and Van Riper (1939) in speech pathology and later, Davis (1947) and Newby (1969) in audiology. Language, and particularly linguistics and psycholinguists, is perhaps still in the formative stage in which the greater share of knowledge is that which is expressed by authorities in the field.

During the age of authorities, the acquisition of knowledge is achieved by referring to relatively well-recognized sources. By this means, an authority may come to represent a school of thought, but the solutions to problems are sometimes complicated by conflicting schools of thought. The school of thought includes not only the views of one or more authorities, but also the interpretation of these views by others. Answers may thus be made up on behalf of certain authorities, as in the statement, "Piaget would answer it this way. . . . "

As the field develops, however, knowledge becomes based more upon verifiable research rather than authoritative observation, and schools of thought tend to give way—sometimes painfully—to conclusions derived through the scientific method. Validity of such conclusions is judged not so much by the identify of the investigator as by the method used to achieve the results.

Mastery of the scientific method has, thus, become the avenue through which one may resolve the dilemmas and the mysteries of his or her professional environment. Although it may assume the ring of a slogan, it must be emphasized at this point that—in a very literal sense—the students of today are the researchers of tomorrow. The unanswered part of the statement is of course, "Which ones?" It is, therefore, imperative for each to try his or her hand at the scientific method in order to assess his or her aptitude and interest as a potential contributor to the knowledge of the field, or at least as an insightful reader of the research from others.

Under optimal conditions, the student's initial exposure to research methodology should be through a comprehensive course in research methods, rather than the thesis experience itself.

An investigative study should become the term project. For the Master's student, as mentioned earlier, the thesis should preferably be optional, based upon both interest and ability. The doctoral student is well-advised to have a realistic dissertation topic chosen and approved by the end of his first year of doctoral study.

TERM PAPER

For the student who is contemplating the research term paper, it may be helpful to realize that the problem-solving activity of research is not really *new*; it is something that one is already doing informally to some extent. The apparent dichotomy between research procedure and clinical practice is not the clear division which it seems. The clinically-oriented student who is contemplating whether or not to try a research project may not realize that the clinical evaluation is, in a sense, a miniature research project, in which the task of the evaluator is to determine which factors are associated with the communication disorder. Screening tests are essentially a matter of determining which children fall within the norm and which are considered outside the normal range. Comparing the diagnostic test results with the expected norms are procedures basically analogous to those used in the more complicated research projects. Finally, the procedures and measures employed to determine whether or not clinical progress was significant contain many essentials of research methodology. In answer to the students' question of whether or not to try to use research methods, it is likely that anyone who tries to test the validity of assumptions or to solve unanswered questions is already using some sort of research method. The formal techniques, however, must be mastered and applied before one's results can stand the test of critical analysis and replication.

THESIS OR DISSERTATION

For the student who is in the contemplative stages of the thesis or dissertation, it will be insightful to view the tentative proposal through the eyes of the faculty advisor. As the student first approaches the potential thesis or dissertation advisor with a general topic, a number of evaluative questions must surely cross the advisor's mind. One of the first is, "How well can the student write?" Although the student has no doubt developed writing skills well enough for adequate answers to examination questions, the demands of research writing call for a more narrative flow, smooth transitions of content, and effective use of compound sentences. Hopefully, a good professional style has been acquired through the composition of term papers. Inasmuch as the advisor is ultimately responsible for the finished work that is handed in it to the graduate school, a writing style composed of short, choppy sentences, informal expressions, and grammatical imprecision, may transform the advisor's editing into unreasonable drudgery.

At a more professional level of interest, the advisor makes a general assessment of the value of the proposed study, through the question, "How well does it fit into the theories and current issues of the discipline?" Although a topic of such as, "The use of the flannel board in articulation therapy", or "A survey of alumni salaries" may have some immediate interest or would give the student some experience in data collecting and writing techniques, they provide little in the way of important theoretical implication or broad application of principles. Related to this general consideration is the potential publishability of the research report. In some cases, where the advisor has a special itnerest in the topic, an arrangement for coauthored publication might be considered. Being unfamiliar with trends in the literature, the student cannot be expected to present an insightful basis for his topic without some guidance, and should also be aware that some topics have more inherent value than others.

"Is this something that the student can really do?", may be the next question in the advisor's mind. For example, some language studies tend to be a statistician's nightmare, with their many subdivisions of variables, and unequal data sets. Audiology, on the other hand, usually fits naturally into a simple research design, with equipment already in routine use and the ready availability of standardized numerical data. In addition to the objective aspects of the proposal, the advisor usually considers how much the student will develop from the experience, whether the scope of the study is too much or too little for the student's capabilities, and other factors, such as whether the procedure will involve the challenge of effective use of instrumentation and statistical techniques.

Finally, the time factor is judged by the advisor's estimate of the difficulties and inconveniences which might be encountered, and weighed against the student's load-organizing ability, and work efficiency. Specifically, a "rush job" never works out according to the student's hopes; the study demands more than the student is prepared to give and sloppy work will never pass. Too much time pressure does not allow for routine contingencies, such as illness of subjects, equipment failure, or scheduling difficulties. The efficient and well-organized student, however, might actually reduce the time anticipated for a graduate degree by taking the thesis option and focusing his efforts on a neat and carefully planned research project.

At this point, the student's curiosity should lead us to the next question, "What would an ideal graduate research study be like?" First, it should be kept simple. Van Riper once advised his students that an ideal research project is to find a group of small things and a group of large things and then show that one is bigger than the other. Of course, there is a bit more to it than that, but the advice is to the point. Complicated studies with indistinct variables are difficult to conduct and awkward to interpret.

There is much to be said about using normal subjects. They are readily available, meet the assumptions of random selection, and allow for careful control of the variables. Clinical cases, on the other hand, do not fit neat criteria, although they tend to be more interesting and to provide topics of more immediate concern to the clinician. From a purely academic point of view, however, most clinical studies fall under the heading of *ex post facto* research (discussed in a later chapter), which has inherent weakness in terms of the researcher's inability to control the independent variable.

Ideally, any equipment used should be standard instrumentation that is already set up in working order. Elaborate hook-ups are impressive but highly prone to failure and, therefore, to delay the project.

The most efficient steppingstone to the review of the literature and to the implementation of effective methodology is the use of a published article or an unpublished thesis or dissertation which has researched a topic closely related to the proposal. An ideal proposal would be readily linked to a well-developed literature from preceding studies. The legacy left by the previous researcher in terms of descriptions, theory, and references was meant to be found and utilized by those who follow.

Practically speaking, few studies meet *all* of the criteria for an ideal experimental design, and those that do are neither necessarily interesting nor widely read. The research endeavor is nearly always a compromise between the content of the project and the efficiency of the design. To take an extreme example, some of the most perfect experiments are conducted on rats, but those in the field of communication disorders would find little of interest or value in such studies because of their remoteness to the human speech process. Stutterers, on the other hand, make notoriously inconsistent research subjects, but warrant continuing research because of the intriguing nature of the disorder.

Not all theses and dissertations must be experimental; there are many other types of research, as described in the next chapter. These include surveys, library studies, inventions, and other contributions which require careful planning and exacting detail, but are not based upon an experimental design. Selection of the most appropriate type of project is usually worked out with one's advisor, and a sound proposal of a nonexperimental nature is perfectly acceptable. The essential point in the preceding discussion is that theses and dissertations are very challenging and sometimes grueling tasks but, for many, they are the key to a learning experience which will continue throughout one's entire career.

CHAPTER 2   Types of Research

Once the general topic for the investigation has been selected, the development of an appropriate experimental method can be a major source of confusion for the student. The concept of a research project may conjure up the image of laboratory equipment, the running of subjects, stacks of computer cards, and large sheets of graphic or numerical data. Depending upon the type of problem to be investigated, however, there is actually a considerable variety of ways in which research may be conducted, with many options for the presentation of results. Many research methods do not rely upon laboratory techniques nor advanced statistical computation. The first step in defining the aim of a research project is to visualize the kind of data to be obtained through the research effort. For example, the data may be in the form of judges' ratings, hearing thresholds, measures from X-ray pictures, test scores, etc. With some notion of the desired data in mind, the method for obtaining the data becomes more apparent. There is, therefore, no particular stereotype to cover all investigative methods; the sort of data needed to answer the research question should dictate the best method to use.

In the pages to follow, some of the more common types of approaches to research problems are discussed. These include experimental investigations, exploratory studies, survey studies, one-subject studies, new technique studies, case studies, and library research. These classifications are not intended to be completely inclusive, nor is it necessarily the best way to classify all types of studies. Many of the categories overlap, so that a specific research project may fit more than one of the descriptions. They are presented in this manner, however, because they tend to be discussed and criticized under these headings, and the classifications provide a convenient way for the student to view his or her own research as well as the research found in the literature. Methodologies and problems typical of the specific areas of the field, i.e., speech pathology, audiology, language, and speech and hearing science, are discussed at the end of the chapter.

EXPERIMENTAL INVESTIGATIONS

This type of investigation is the most common approach to research found in current literature relating to the speech and hearing areas. Most experimental investigations originate from an observation or belief that seems to be true, but that has never been demonstrated in a systematic way. For example, nearly everyone who has listened to a recording of his or her own voice has

9

the initial impression that the voice sounds a bit strange; most of us think that our "real" voice might sound better or more "natural" than the recording, and persons with voice problems are often reluctant to change their pitch or quality beause their habitual speech seems more natural. In an experiment to test the validity of this clinical observation, eleven young adult males were asked to compare fundamental frequencies of their own live and recorded voices with those of the rest of the group (Haskell and Baker, 1978). It was found that individuals were accurate in judging the fundamental frequency of all recorded voices, but were not accurate in judging the sound of their own live voice. In other words, we always tend to hear our own voice as being "average", regardless of its actual characteristics. The study verified the clinical observation that voice patients fail to perceive their own vocal anomalies. As another example to test a clinical observation, there is a rather common assumption among clinicians that vocal nodules can usually be detected by listening to the voice. An experimental investigation, however, revealed that the majority of such evaluations are actually incorrect, and that experienced clinicians are no more accurate than graduate students in detecting the presence of nodules (Dice and Shearer, 1973).

In addition to the verification or negation of common assumptions, the experimental investigation usually reveals additional—sometimes unexpected—results that point the way toward new avenues of research. In this way, the pursuit of research answers is never final because new evidence nearly always raises new questions.

As a general rule, the experimental method of investigation tends to be more efficient than some of the other approaches, because the subjects to be investigated can be carefully selected and control procedures can be introduced into the project so as to eliminate unwanted influences in the results. Also—unless an elaborate series of variables are involved—the efficiency of the method allows for a rather compact style of reporting, as compared for instance, with library research. Finally, because of the standardization under which this type of study is conducted, it is quite feasible to plan the entire project with sufficient detail to set up an accurate timetable for the completion of each phase. The most efficient investigations involve relatively few variables, with each variable being precisely defined, and an overall experimental design that is based upon simplicity. In the case of graduate student research, these factors should be covered as much as possible in the prospectus stages of the project, so that possible areas of difficulty can be anticipated and resolved in advance.

In the strictest sense of the definition, experimental research means that the independent variable is controlled by the experimenter, in order to measure its effect upon the dependent variable. By this definition, many clinical studies are not strictly experimental. For instance, if the speech of aphasics is to be the independent variable (with audience response as the dependent variable), the experimenter must assume that the aphasics are good typical examples of the intended variable. In other words, the fact that a research study employed an experimental design and the use of statistics does not, in itself, indicate an *experimental investigation*, unless the experimenter can control all of the main variables. Although an experimental investigation is sometimes considered to be the highest form of research, it is by no means the only acceptable type, and the most appropriate mode of research is the one that best fits the problem and the situation available.

EXPLORATORY STUDIES

The most efficient examples of experimental investigations, as discussed earlier, are those in which nothing goes unplanned. At times, however, the experimenter is interested in a topic for which there is little or no background and, therefore, little basis for precise planning. The whole point of the study in this case is a venture into the unknown, looking into an entirely new phenomenon that does not relate directly to any previous line of research. An exploratory study, therefore,, has certain disadvantages, in that the investigative method will be tried in unforseen circumstances, giving little assurance that the method will work or that it will really measure what the investigator is trying to study.

When there are many uncertainties in the method and the type of data to be anticipated, a few subjects (three to five or more, if subjects are plentiful) are run through the procedure in order to see what kinds of difficulties might arise. This technique is termed a "pilot study" because it is used as a guide to plot the course for the main project that is to follow. Although the pilot study is particularly valuable in the exploratory type of study, it is sometimes treated as a routine first step in any major investigation. "Pilot data" are also considered essential for most studies in which research grants may sponsor the work.

From the standpoint of the student, exploratory studies pose a rather pragmatic problem in assembling a scholarly review of the literature for a thesis or dissertation. Sparce availability of direct references, however, should not imply that the review of the literature will be superficially presented, rather that the references will probably be drawn from a broader base and that their application to the present study must be more fully explained.

The exploratory study, as a rule, does not intend to probe too deeply into a topic, but is designed rather to show that a certain characteristic exists and can be identified. It may call attention to the importance and research possibilities of an area that has been previously ignored. The importance of an exploratory investigation is, therefore, to point the way toward future research, and to stimulate other studies to follow. In theses and dissertations, the title itself may indicate the exploratory nature of the study, as shown by "An Exploratory Investigation of _____." In journal articles, however, titles run somewhat shorter and the exploratory or "preliminary study" designation is not often used. When the topic has been researched beyond the initial stages, its investigation no longer has an exploratory nature. Studies dealing with a heavily researched area, such as the adaptation effect in stuttering, for example, could hardly be considered exploratory because of the wealth of material available from previous investigations. The experimental designs, procedures, common variables, and appropriate statistics for conducting studies in adaptation have already been reported in the literature. On the other hand, research into an area such as differences in auditory perception among persons with normal hearing has never received much attention, and study into this topic would contain many uncertainties and might require some initial trial and error because of its exploratory nature.

SURVEY STUDIES

When the topic to be investigated deals with the attitudes, opinions, characteristics, or experiences of relatively large groups, the survey method is used. The most common example of the survey method is found in Speech Pathology, in which surveys are made to determine the incidence of various speech disorders among certain age groups or other populations. Senturia and Wilson (1968) for example, found the incidence of voice disorders in a large group of school children to be about 6%. Another survey of the clinical records from over four thousand residents in a special state school revealed the incidence of stuttering to be approximately 5% of the mentally retarded population (Schaeffer and Shearer, 1968).

In circumstances where the population is less accessible, a random sample can be selected to represent the larger group. In a study based upon a random sample of 162 clients enrolled in speech therapy from a wide variety of clinics, it was reported that from the client's point of view, the physical appearance of the clinician was least important, while technical skill seemed to be the most important factor related to clinical progress (Haynes and Oratio, 1978). In this case, the 162 clients are assumed to represent a much larger population. Other survey topics have included types of case load among school speech clinicians, evaluation of training programs by alumni, public attitudes toward speech and hearing problems, and language test scores from different ethnic groups of school children. As one might surmise from the variety of topics, the survey method can take many forms, varying from a mailed questionnaire to the interviewing or testing of clinical populations.

Surveys conducted by mail are only as effective as the form provided for the subjects' response, and a one- or two-page checklist stands a much better chance of return than does a five-page list of complicated items. A cover letter should accompany the questionnaire, explaining briefly the purpose of the survey, the investigator's thanks and appreciation for the reply, and an offer to send a summary of the results upon request. A self-addressed envelope should also be enclosed for returning the completed form.

Generally speaking, a return from more than one-half of the correspondents would be considered a fairly representative sample, while two-thirds or more would be considered very good. Depending upon the type of population to be surveyed, a return of even one-third is sometimes entirely adequate. In the study mentioned earlier, surveying the factors in clinical progress, a rather ambitious effort was made to obtain responses from a national sample of clients receiving speech therapy. One hundred clinical settings were contacted for the distribution of questionnaires to their clients (Haynes and Oratio, 1978). From a distribution of 500 questionnaires, 162 were returned, yielding a response of 32.4% to the survey. The response, however, represented a wide geographical area, several types of clinical settings, all types of speech disorders, and an age range from ten to eighty years. Sample populations from individuals who feel a professional obligation to respond or have a need to be heard from are most likely to yield a high percentage of returns. Groups of this nature have included public school speech clinicians, clinical audiologists, and alumni from certain university training programs.

In addition to surveys conducted by mail or through the analysis of case histories and similar records, many surveys are based upon a personal interview with individuals from a certain population. In one university, for example, all entering freshmen were asked if they had ever stuttered as a child (Shearer and Williams, 1965). All who responded affirmatively (58 subjects) were interviewed individually in order to study the circumstances under which stuttering behavior had subsequently disappeared.

Although most surveys in the speech and hearing areas are based upon people, some are based upon objects, physical facilities, or techniques used in various settings. If the items to be surveyed are considered to be consistent and highly representative of a larger population, a very small sample may be sufficient. Only nine clinical facilities were included in a survey to check for the presence of bacteria in stock earmolds used in hearing testing (Lankford and Behnke, 1973). Earmold cleaning methods were found to be uniformly adequate and consistent among all types of facilities in the sample.

The results of surveys are usually reported descriptively, that is by means of charts, graphs, and tables, rather than in the form of statistical significance alone. Percentages and proportions are particularly suited for the descriptive reporting of survey data, as typified in the Lankford and Behnke (1973) survey: "Although 20 of the 36 earmolds harbored some type of bacteria, the quantities of bacteria isolated were very small and probably less than would be expected . . . "

ONE-SUBJECT STUDIES

Because the letter N is used in statistical formulas to denote the number of subjects in an experiment, it has become a standard symbol in discuisng sample size, as it might apply to methods and results. Terms such as "large N" and "small N" tell us something about the nature of an experiment. An "N-of-one" study is one in which the results were based upon the performance of only one subject. The rationale for single-subject studies is, of course, that the subject is representative of a large population, and that one trained subject who is tested in depth will provide more complete information than would a group of subjects tested less definitively. In other instances, there may be only one subject available who fits a certain category, as in the case of a patient with a certain type of implanted hearing aid or other unique classification. Reich and Lerman (1978), for example, reported the laboratory analysis of the voice from one patient who had undergone teflon injection treatment for a paralyzed vocal cord. Experimental results from one subject, however, should be distinguished from a *case study*, which is usually a descriptive report of the diagnosis and clinical progress of a client with a certain type of disorder or special therapy.

Some examples of one-subject research are conducted under circumstances where the nature of the task demands a dedication or motivation that cannot be expected from a general group of subjects. Particularly difficult or precise tasks may require a period of special training or special capabilities in the subject. These procedures might include difficult phonatory exercises for the recording of muscle activity, or skilled listening for detailed acoustic stimuli.

Optimally, the choice of the subject for study should be made on the basis of some a priori information about what might constitute a typical or an atypical individual. These indications could be derived from related research or from the previous experience of the investigator. Inspection of the literature dealing with activity of the normal speech mechanism, including movements of structures, air flow and pressure changes, and electromyographic measures, usually reveals many exceptions to the normative pattern. It is often seen that as many as two of five subjects do not quite fit the modal display from the rest of the group. Because most studies are based upon general trends and statistical averages, exceptions to the rule are not necessarily brought out in the results. Shipp (1975), however, illustrates individual differences among six subjects in a study of laryngeal movement. He notes that the larynx rises with increased fundamental frequency in four subjects, but shows an exceptional downward trend in two subjects. One may assume, therefore, that the odds would be two-to-one in favor of choosing a typically representative subject of this type of one-subject study, but the risk of measuring an atypical example should always be taken into consideration. From a practical standpoint, although one-subject studies are perfectly legitimate, they are not frequently used; studies that are designed to incorporate the smallest possible N nearly always report data based upon four to eight subjects.

Finally, as a resut of recently implemented federal regulations involving the use of human subjects for research purposes, researchers have encountered major limitations in the use of techniques such as X-ray photography, electric shock conditioning, tranquilizing drugs, and implanted electrodes. Briefly, these regulations (discussed in a later chapter) prohibit the use of any technique or procedure deemed hazardous to anyone who serves as a subject in a research project. The long range influence of these restrictions will severely curtail some types of investigations, and in other instances, may force the investigator to use himself as the only available subject.

STUDIES TO DEMONSTRATE NEW TECHNIQUES

Reports which describe new techniques, new methods, new tests, or new inventions appear rather frequently in the literature. Many of the reports are simply to describe the way in which a new piece of equipment or test method may be assembled and used. The theory under which the new device is developed and used is also included in most of these reports. Depending upon the type of supportive material used in the report, the presentation of a new technique may or may not be considered to be investigative research. Fletcher et al. (1975), for example, reported the development and use of instrumentation for displaying continuous computer-generated palatograms. The report simply described and illustrated the technique and recommended its use as a research instrument. The report appeared as a relatively brief search note. In other examples, the new technique is described in conjunction with its use as the method in an experimental investigation. Using this approach, a new technique for measuring tongue motion by means of light sensors was demonstrated in a study on the coarticulation of consonants with Chinese vowels (Chuang and Wang, 1978). This type of presentation, in a sense, carries the new technique report one step further through the addition of a research topic with experimental method and results. Analogous new techniques may be found in terms of test batteries or programmed learning packages for use in articulation, audiology, and language. Particularly in the children's language development area, the field has experienced a remarkable increase in evaluative testing materials and procedures.

The development of new techniques in the form of instrumentation, tests, programs, etc., contributes greatly to the technology of the field and represents a research area that may be overlooked as an appropriate venture for a thesis or dissertation.

CASE STUDIES

The case study is another type of report that may or may not be viewed as research, depending upon how the study is conducted and reported. As a general rule, the description of one or more clinical cases, along with the therapy and the outcome of clinical mangement contains few elements of research. Although such reports have a high degree of practical value and often provide insight and the sharing of professional thought, they do not necessarily contribute new knowledge.

As in the studies that involve the implementation of new techniques, the case study is sometimes expanded to include an experimental hypothesis, research procedure, and objective results. The procedures may involve approaches to therapy, diagnostic classifications, behavioral observations, or prognostic clues to clinical results. In a case study involving a 61-year-old male whose dysphonia from vocal cord paralysis was improved by teflon injection, periodic speech samples were recorded over a one-year period. Analysis of variance revealed significant improvements in listeners' evaluations of the voice over the recovery period (Reich and Lerman, 1978). Acoustical analyses were also made for comparisons between speech samples. As a result of the study, the authors pointed out the need for quantifiable measures in evaluation and periodic assessment of clinical cases. In this study, a research question was asked and a conclusion drawn from the data.

LONGITUDINAL AND CROSS-SECTIONAL STUDIES

An investigative method that is uniquely suited to developmental or progressive clinical phenomena is the longitudinal study. Basically, the principle of the longitudinal study is to observe or retest the *same individuals* over a period of time, instead of testing a different group at each age level. The most obvious example is in child development, in which a single group of children would be tested for articulation or language acquisition over a period of, say, three years. The more common alternative would be to test three separate groups of children—one group at each age level. This latter method is called the *cross-sectional* approach.

The essential feature of the longitudinal study—the time span—makes this approach inadvisable for most graduate student endeavors, because a data collection process requiring more than one year would be unrealistic in many graduate degree programs. Although one year or less might be adequate for observing some types of developmental trends, longitudinal studies must sometimes be based upon trends over several years rather than several months.

From the standpoint of research design, the longitudinal study is considered to be superior to the cross-sectional groups method, both in terms of reliability and validity. In other words, a duplication of the study would be more likely to yield the same results, and the procedure is more likely to measure the intended characteristic.

This advantage is achieved by the fact that the original group is retained for the measures at each developmental stage; no new groups are selected. When cross-sectional groups are used to show each developmental stage, the inherent weakness lies in the possibility that the groups might simply be different from each other, and the study is not really measuring development at all. As an illustration, let us say that an investigator finds 15% of the first grade children in a school district to be delayed in language. He or she finds no language delay among the high school seniors, and concludes that language problems improve completely between grade one and grade twelve. The weakness, as suggested in the preceding discussion, is that the high school seniors may be an entirely different type of person from the first graders, and that the language problems could have gotten worse instead of better, to the point where the language disordered children have dropped out of school. Thus, either of the two opposing conclusions could be drawn from the results. The potential error which is avoided in the longitudinal study is called the error of *group selectivity*.

The nemesis of longitudinal research is attrition of the sample size with the passage of time. People move away, die, lost interest, or otherwise miss the testing dates before the study can be completed. For this reason, longitudinal studies tend to be expensive, in that extra travel, correspondence, phone calls, and payment to subjects may be involved in keeping the data sample intact. To some extent, a carefully matched subject may be substituted occasionally when one is lost from the study group, but this practice is to be avoided as much as possible. A secondary factor that sometimes influences longitudinal research is an environmental change that could effect the course of development. For instance, if an earthquake, flood, fire, loss of funds, or political dispute, were to close the schools for an extended period, the test scores might show poor development for that time. Finally, the subjects in a longitudinal study tend to become test-educated from repeated testing over a period of time, so that the experimental procedure itself may actually be responsible for improved test scores. For this reason, the investigator should reveal as little as possible to the subjects about the tests or scoring criteria.

In summary, the strengths and weaknesses of longitudinal research are compared typically to those of the cross-sectional approach for the study of development. The longitudinal approach is considered to be stronger in reliability and validity, in that the same group is followed over time. Because the subjects are always compared with themselves, the group "matching" is perfect, but the method is cumbersome and often expensive. Its potential weaknesses are in attrition of subjects, unusual environmental influences, and testing sophistication. The cross-sectional approach has the advantage of being efficient and relatively quick in administration. It is also relatively immune to subject attrition, environmental factors, and testing sophistication. Its major weakness is in the possibility that the results could be attributible to biased selection of the cross-sectional groups. Most reference sources consider the longitudinal approach to be by far the stronger type of design. Campbell and Stanley (1963), however, point out that from a completely idealistic point of view, a combination of the two approaches would counterbalance the weakness in each design. Realistically, however, neither the combination design nor the longitudinal method are within the feasible limitations of every investigator, and the cross-sectional approach is, therefore, the more practical choice.

Not all longitudinal studies are developmental in the maturational sense; some are designed to plot the course of a progressive pathology, such as multiple sclerosis, or to evaluate the improvement in disorders such as aphasia and laryngectomy. In its most simplified form, the longitudinal study is an elaboration on the pretest-posttest type of investigation, in which a group of subjects is tested before and after therapy, surgery, or other influential event. The term "longitudinal", however, usually implies the use of periodic testing which may extend through several months or years.

It is an unfortunate paradox that the professional group that is most conveniently situated to conduct longitudinal research—the school speech clinicians—is usually the least likely to become involved in such ambitious research endeavors. The general nature of most school environments does not allow the time nor provide the incentive to pursue research projects of a major magnitude. Topics that might be applied in the school situation could include 'Factors Associated with the Development or Reduction of Non-fluency in Children", "Characteristics of Children who do and do not Self-Improve Articulation Errors", or "Language Development in Children with Chronic Otitis Media".

LIBRARY RESEARCH

This method of investigation is more commonly found in the typically literary fields such as English literature, speech communication, history, and philosophy, rather than in communication disorders or speech and hearing science. Library studies are usually involved with historical trends, or with the development of certain concepts, organizations, or social influences. Others may summarize a specific topic, sometimes in an authoritative type of review entitled, "The State of the Art." Such articles are often written at the request of a journal editor who wishes to present a summary from the viewpoint of a recognized scholar in the field. Regardless of the topic or style of presentation, the library study is typically based upon some central theme that the investigator wishes to trace through the literature.

Library research studies of a historical nature are not particularly common in the speech and hearing areas, perhaps because the field itself is relatively new and few topics would be suited to a detailed historical review. The American Speech and Hearing Association was founded about 50 years ago, and Audiology as a discipline did not develop until World War II. The communication disorders topic with the oldest documented history in the United States is the development of schools for the deaf, rather than the broader field that we know today. More typically, literary work in this field is based upon discussions of an argumentative rather than historical nature, as in the following:

Ramp, D., and Pennbacker, M., Indications and Contraindications for Tongue Thrust Therapy. *Lang. Speech Hearing Serv. Schools*, 9, 254–258, 1978.

Franks, J., and Daniloff, R., A Review of the Audiological Implications of Testing Vowel Perception. *J. Aud. Res.*, 13, 355–368, 1973.

Sheehan, J., and Costley, M., A Reexammination of the Role of Heredity in Stuttering. *J. Speech Hearing Dis.*, 42, 47–59, 1977.

The seeds of a library study may often be found in a published bibliography on some specific topic. An intriguing presentation of this nature is a brief article by Trotter and Silverman (1976), entitled "The Stutterer as a Character in Contemporary Literature: A Bibliography."

Access to a very complete library is, of course, critical to the success of this type of study, because it assumes that all of the important relevant information will be included and documented in a fully comprehensive presentation. Theses and dissertations of this type are, therefore, inclined to be considerably longer than those involving a single laboratory project. In view of the comprehensive nature of the work, it is important to define the scope of the investigation as to the number of years to be covered, and which specific aspects of the topic will and will not be included.

In a sense, nearly every example of published research contains a miniature library study as part of the introductory section which refers to related research. More extensive reviews of the literature commonly comprise the second chapter of theses and dissertations.

CHAPTER 3

Characteristics of Specific Research Areas: Speech Pathology, Language, Audiology, and Speech and Hearing Science

Within any field of study, some broad generalizations can be made as to the sorts of problems most commonly encountered in research and the investigative strategies that are most often employed in that discipline. In experimental psychology, for instance, we are all familiar with the use of laboratory rats or of large numbers of students from the introductory classes who serve as subjects. Typical experimental projects might involve motor ability, perception, or learning, with the results computed from a randomized block design. Within the communication sciences, each specialty area is geared toward a different aspect of the communication process, and each tends to have its own variables and strategies uniquely suited for solving its research problems. For example, many studies in experimental phonetics are based upon measures from the three vowels: /i/, /a/, and /u/; audiological research projects often incorporate the pure tone frequencies between 500 and 2000 Hz; and language development studies frequently compare the linguistic patterns of different ethnic groups and different age levels. Although some general characterizations could hardly encompass the whole thrust of research in each area, it provides a better understanding and appreciation of the research efforts in different parts of the field. Particularly for the graduate student, some impression of the characteristics and scope of research topics within a given professional area should enhance one's ability to formulate appropriate questions and to find suitable models from which to develop a plan of investigation. Before embarking on an expedition, it is helpful to get a general picture of the territory.

SPEECH PATHOLOGY

Research in speech pathology covers a broader and more diverse area than does audiology or language, and deals heavily in clinical concepts that are subjective and that do not have an inherent numerical value. Although test

19

scores are well-suited to statistical treatment, evaluative terms such as *degree* of severity, *rate* of improvement, *level* of motivation, or *effectiveness* of therapy are matters of clinical judgment that must be transformed into numbers before statistics can be applied. The process of numerical conversion usually takes one of two forms: defined classifications or judges' ratings. Defined classifications are those that assign numerical value to a condition according to certain definitions. In voice disorders, for instance, we may find a "number two vocal closure" or a "number three nasality", as defined by certain criteria. The reliability of defined classifications depends upon the degree of objectivity that can be used in the criteria. Judges' ratings of severity or quality of the speech sample are usually based on a seven-point scale, with a descriptive term to indicate the two opposite extremes of the scale. In many forms of judges' ratings, several descriptive areas are applied to each speech sample. These might include pleasant-unpleasant, clear-unclear, effective-ineffective, etc. An alternative method of judges' ratings is one in which each judge arranges all samples in rank order from highest to lowest degree of the characteristic being evaluated. Ten speech samples, for instance, might be lined up according to intelligibility, from best to poorest, based upon the judges' impressions.

The numerical values for the effectiveness of some types of therapy are derived from the number of trials or the number of minutes needed to reach each achievement level. This technique is especially suited to programmed learning packages available for articulation therapy.

A very simple rating scale for articulation performance was used by Stephens and Daniloff (1977), who incorporated the judgments of three experienced clinicians to score children's /s/ productions on a three-point scale. Ratings were −1 (unacceptable), +1 (acceptable), and 0 (uncertain).

Perhaps one reason for the early proliferation of adaptation studies to chart the reduction of stuttering is that this basic design is fairly predictable in producing organized statistical data. A dissertation or thesis on this topic can be reasonably assured of having a clearly defined statistical result. However, even the data yielded from counting the number of blocks from the oral readings of a paragraph have a subjective aspect, which must sometimes be resolved by having several judges agree on the correct tally.

Other relatively standard approaches to research in speech pathology may be found in the test-retest method for evaluating improvement in speech therapy, or in the reporting of standardized test results administered to a certain clinical group. Where feasible, these methods should include the testing of a control group for comparative measures.

Substantial research in articulation deals with the normative achievement of articulation skills at various age levels. Because speech development is influenced by many factors in addition to age, close attention must be paid to matching each age group according to sex, I.Q., hearing, and home or school environment. Other research efforts in articulation have been in comparing the differences among several commercial tests, as well as test scores obtained from different types of speech samples, such as imitative, spontaneous, or oral reading. These studies are often evaluative, with conclusions relating to the efficiency, effectiveness, and other comparative merits of the test instruments. As in other types of communicative disorders, occasional studies in articulation are centered upon basic sensory, psychological, or physiological weaknesses that might account for the presence of articulatory anomalies. Such studies may investigate areas such as tactile discrimination of the oral structures or acoustic discrimination of various speech cues.

Voice disorders are often reported in the form of case studies or as illustrative examples of certain clinical methodologies, which are primarily in discussion form, and do not necessarily use statistical results. Specific variations in vocal production are usually studied in the speech science laboratory, where the acoustic or physiological aspects are analyzed through instrumental methods. These are usually reported by means of descriptive statistics, which involve mainly the presentation of percentages, or of charts showing physiological changes for different pitches or qualities.

LANGUAGE

A comparatively new area of investigation is Language. The importance of this aspect of communication disorders cannot be overemphasized; in a recent survey of speech clinicians in Illinois (Williams, 1977), 95 percent of those responding indicated that their first choice of professional interest was in children's language development. As a research area, however, much of the normative data have not yet been established and many investigators, therefore, tend to cram too many research questions into one study. The typical language study may involve two or more groups of children, three or more sampling conditions, and from four to sixteen linguistic categories to be assessed. The picture may be even further complicated by the addition of other elements, such as item analysis of the test battery, parental responses, parental language patterns, consistency of errors, and differences in listener agreement. From a statistical standpoint, the language study is thus plagued by a multitude of variables, partial factors, and confounding influences that do not always fit an efficient experimental design.

Because of the myriad of questions to be answered, the statistical approach must be broad enough in scope to include multiple results. Some form of multivatiate analysis, such as multiple regression or discriminate function, is representative of a class of statistics that can handle many variables at the same time, and this approach has been utilized effectively in some language studies. In a study involving children's comprehension strategies (Chapman and Kohn, 1978), a multiple regression analysis was used to assess the effects of age, mean length of utterance (MLU), and short term memory (STM) on comprehension performance. Included in the procedure and analysis were three age groups, 36 sentences, seven categories of responses, and five types of comprehension strategies. As one might expect, the classic research model of one independent variable and one dependent variable would hardly cover the many relationships to be presented in the results and discussion.

The multivariate statistical approach, which requires a computer program is perhaps the most efficient way to handle this type of interrelated data, but the sophistication of this kind of analysis and the interpretation of results is often beyond the student's grasp. Standard computer programs available for data groups of this nature include stepwise multiple regression, discriminate analysis, Hotelling's T-test, and multivariate analysis of variance.

At the opposite end of the treatment continuum is what might be termed the segmental approach to bringing out the results from a large and interrelated data pile. Through this technique, each question or part of the hypothesis is brought up separately and treated more or less on an individual basis, using either descriptive statistics or group comparisons. In some cases, a rather large project may be divided into a series of smaller studies, with each devoted to a particular part of the major topic. An article that addressed a series of research questions, using relatively simple but effective statistical techniques explored the relationships between some aspects of language development and sensorimotor development (Folger and Leonard, 1978). Variables included types of children, stages of language skills, age, sensorimotor development, and differences in testing scales. Measures of interest were compared by the use of several Mann-Whitney U tests and rank order correlations. This method tends to spread the results out into separate headings as compared to tying it together into a single package by the use of a multiple-factor type of statistic. The segmental treatment of results, however, has some advantage in helping the reader to visualize each part, and in the case of student research it provides a natural outline for the arrangement of the points to be considered in the study.

A third approach is perhaps a compromise between the two types of treatments just described. Basically, this involves putting the main factors into an analysis of variance, and then treating each additional point by a simpler computational method. This approach can usually be worked on a calculator, and still has the advantage of testing for interaction effects between the main variables.

As research in the language field evolves, its territory will become more familiar to its investigators and many of its factors will become known to the point where fewer influences need be considered in a single study. Thus, as the field matures, its development will probably be toward less complicated experimental designs, and toward the use of more well-tried methods, which will come eventually through common use, to be considered as standard procedures.

Language as a Basic Concept in Speech and Hearing

Although all of the separate disciplines within the Speech and Hearing Sciences tend to overlap in content and general concepts, the discipline known as Language seems to reach into associated areas more readily than the rest. The origins of language research developed as a rather narrowly limited study of language development in children. However, speech clinicians who were working with articulation began to believe that proper pronunciation of individual phonemes did not quite seem to describe the whole process faced by the misarticulating child. The answer seemed to lie more in the formative aspects of the total speech output—in the child's language.

With what seemed to be the "discovery" of an area known as language pathology, new avenues of research began to blossom immediately. In keeping with its origins, which were closely allied with articulation, language soon become the dominating aspects of children's remedial speech, and the concepts of speech development have now been largely superseded by what is called language development. Within the area of children's speech therapy, articulation has now come to be treated as a subdivision of language. Panagos and his associates (Panagos and King, 1975; Matheny and Panagos, 1978; Schmauch et al., 1978; Panagos et al., 1979) have exemplified the inseparable relationship between language and articulation, and the value of viewing articulation disorders through language research.

Strangely, the more formal science of linguistics has remained somewhat divorced and perhaps even aloof from what is commonly known as language, as it is applied in our field. The research in linguistics is often considered to be remote, abstract, and frequently composed of little more than authoratative viewpoints. Supportive research for linguistic theories has tended to be uneven, and the area has maintained its posture as somewhat of a philosophy, with only an indirect application to clinical problems.

Language development and language pathology have gradually begun to expand even beyond the boundaries of articulation. Some years ago, Soderberg (1967) along with Bloodstein and Gantwerk (1967), reported on the utilization of language concepts in explaining the location and severity of stuttering blocks. More recently, Adams and Ramig (1980) and Riley and Riley (1980) have described stuttering behavior related to the complexity of language formation patterns, leading the study of language further into the clinical aspects of stuttering. Similarly, syntactic principles have appeared as part of the test batteries for the evaluation and predictive characteristics of asphasia (Brookshire and Nicholas, 1980). The field of learning disabilities has been heavily saturated with the concepts of language, to the point where language has formed common ground between the fields of Speech Pathology and Special Education.

In deaf education and rehabilitation of hearing impaired, the advancing familiarity with sign language has just begun to incorporate the fundamentals of language research as a valuable tool in comprehending the learning strategies for complex sign patterns. The influence of sign language skills upon the development of syntactic abilities in deaf children has also been reported (Brasel and Quigley, 1977). In audiology, the role of language comprehension as an influence in speech discrimination represents an additional avenue for future research.

In summary, the continuing trend in language is to enter other aspects of the field of communication disorders and to form a common base for the field in general. Students who are developing research interests along with clinical skills in nearly any part of the field would seem well-advised to develop a good grounding in the principles of language and language development, because these concepts may serve in the comprehension of many allied specializations.

AUDIOLOGY

For simplicity of experimental design, the field of audiology lends itself particularly well to research methodology. Hearing testing is essentially the process of assigning numerical values to the client's hearing ability. In most cases, these values are in the form of auditory thresholds recorded in decibels or speech discrimination scores in percentages. Sample populations, for the most part, can be well-defined and classified as to their hearing capability or by the medical diagnosis of their hearing pathology. An additional advantage is that research instrumentation is readily available in the form of the standardized test equipment that is used and calibrated routinely for clinical audiology.

Many studies in audiology are well-suited to a three-factor analysis of variance, involving the factors: types of subjects, test conditions, and hearing stimuli. This rather common design can be seen in the initial part of a study to test the reliability of the comfort loudness setting in hearing aids. An analysis of variance was computed for two types of subjects (experienced and inexperienced hearing aid users), two test conditions (two comfort settings), and three hearing stimuli (three hearing aids) (Walden *et al.*, 1977). Simpler studies in this area often involve only a comparison of two sets of data, such as hearing thresholds before and after noise exposure, or hearing performance with two different types of hearing aids.

Much of the research in audiology can be seen in terms of trends that follow each new technological advancement in the field, such as the Bekesy audiometer, the evoked response averaging computer, and the impedance bridge. As each new technique is brought forth, an accompanying series of research studies can usually be predicted as a means of answering the many new clinical questions generated.

SPEECH AND HEARING SCIENCE

Studies in speech and hearing science are devoted mainly to finding new information about the structures and workings of the normal speech and hearing process. The results of these studies may or may not have clinical implications; their main contribution is toward basic research. Research in speech and hearing science is usually conducted under laboratory conditions and is characterized by well-defined variables and a neatness in experimental design. Subjects are usually selected on the basis of normal speech and hearing in order to provide a relatively homogeneous group. Purists in the speech science area are sometimes even reluctant to extend their scope of research into speech pathology because the lack of uniformity in clinical populations may serve to "contaminate" an otherwise carefully controlled study.

From a disinterested viewpoint, the dicotomy between research in speech science and in speech pathology is remarkable, because both are concerned essentially with the same processes and concepts. However, the speech scientist, as mentioned previously, does not wish to compromise his laboratory methodology by dealing with the uncertain qualities of clinical cases. The clinician, on the other hand, typically comes ill-prepared for scientific methodology because clinical training has naturally emphasized the pathologies, and students tend to steer clear of extra courses in speech science, experimental phonetics, statistics, acoustics, and experimental methodology. As a result of the strong divergence in the two philosophies, research in speech has come to be polarized under two independent headings. The result is an unfortunate lack of sharing between speech science and speech pathology. A notable exception may be found, however, in the area of cleft palate, in which clinicians tend to maintain a research-oriented approach to the pathology.

Research in hearing science and audiology has maintained a close interrelationship, to the point where no clear division is recognized between the two branches of the discipline. As a group, audiologists tend to keep up their background in anatomy, physiology, acoustics, and other aspects of hearing science, even though their responsibilities may be entirely clinical. By the same token, most hearing science research into the characteristics of the normal ear carries some direct and helpful contributions to better clinical insight.

Statistically, speech and hearing science is too broad an area to be described by any typical pattern. If anything, the statistical treatments in this area are inclined to be extremely simple, drawing heavily upon descriptive results which may be presented as percentages, means, and standard deviations. Because many psychophysical studies are based upon very small Ns, results from each subject are sometimes described individually rather than summarized in terms of group averages.

CHAPTER 4

Realistic Considerations for the Research Project

Particularly with graduate student research, an initial planning stage is imperative in order to insure the feasibility of the study and to invite some advising, editing, and modifications of the proposal. This process of assistance is usually conducted in a prospectus (or preprospectus) meeting. (See the section on the prospectus outline.) Before the investigation is actually begun, the following points should be considered thoughtfully and incorporated into the overall plan:

1. What is the importance of the study?
2. Will the methodology effectively show a result?
3. What type of data will be produced, and how will it be evaluated?
4. Are the subjects available in the type and quantity needed?
5. Will the proposed sample of data adequately represent the population?
6. Is the proper equipment (if required) available and functional?
7. Can the study be completed in the allotted period of time?

1. IMPORTANCE OF THE STUDY

The importance of the study is the most subjective aspect of the proposal, and one that cannot be predicted with complete accuracy. Ultimately, the importance of any research is a matter of how well it fills a gap in some body of information. This can be determined roughly by how often it is referenced and also by how it is supported by subsequent research. By this criterion, importance cannot be judged until some time after the results of the study are published. The most outstanding examples of important published work are sometimes referred to as "classic" studies. Studebaker's (1964) research on the most effective use of masking noise in hearing testing, or Hollien's (1960) X-ray analysis of vocal cord thickness during changes in pitch are referenced as the basis for many other studies, and could perhaps be considered as classics by this standard.

Good suggestions, complete with rationale, for future studies are sometimes provided by the discussion sections of journal articles, in which the author speculates on topics which seem to be the next logical link in the chain of his investigations. Reviewing a few articles in the student's interest area should, therefore, be an effective and convenient way to gain some direction in the planning of significant research proposals. Review of even a relatively small number of articles on a given topic will usually enable one to compile a list of insightful research questions. Here are a few examples:

"The middle (Evoked Response Audiometry) responses may be of secondary reliance, but further study is needed to determine their applicability in situations involving young individuals or sedation."

(Skinner and Glattke, 1977, p. 196)

"The nature of the role of comprehension processing strategies used by listeners in the sentence elicited imitation task merit further investigation."

(Hudgens and Culliman, 1978, p. 818)

"Future studies providing clearer descriptions of the specific types of disfluent behaviors that are reinforced or punished may clarify some of the confusion surrounding this issue."

(Daly and Kimbarow, 1978, p. 596)

Importance, however, is a very relative concept, and what appears as a trivial detail at the moment may assume considerable importance when the time comes to fit this small building block into a later construct. The graduate student engaged in basic research is sometimes intimidated by questions as to what purpose will be served by the results of the study. Grant Fairbanks, who was one of the pioneers in speech science advised his students never to apologize about their research because it had no apparent application; if it could add something to our understanding, it would be worthwhile.

2. EFFECTIVENESS OF THE METHODOLOGY

A practical question that underlies the whole study is, "Will the method work?" Most of the uncertainties can be answered by conducting a small pilot study using from one to five subjects in order to discover potential weaknesses in the procedures. Even in the early planning stage, the methodology should be described in enough detail to allow a realistic evaluation of its feasibility. In some cases, for example, the test battery should be cut so as to reduce subject fatigue; in others, the proposed tests may not be sensitive enough to distinguish between important differences.

Some of the more frequent deficiencies in proposed methodology include:

1. The proposal is too ambitious and unwieldy. Too many variables are included, or the study is based on running too many types of subjects, making too many spectrograms, or subjecting listeners to too many samples.

2. A control group is not used in a study for which the clinical sample should be compared with a normal population.

3. Instructions to subjects are poorly defined or leave room for confusion ad variability of performance.

4. The tabulation or measurement method will not produce uniform results and there is no provision to establish reliability of the data.

Indirectly related to the effectiveness of the design and methodology is the concept of "salvage value" for the project as a whole. Salvage value refers to the potential value of the conclusions, regardless of how the results may turn out. Particularly for student research, the optimum arrangement is one in which either significance or nonsignificance of the statistical results will yield an answer to the research question. Although the mature investigator can afford to try some studies that serve only to test the feasibility of a methodology or general concept, the thesis word or dissertation should be constructed tightly enough to allow for acceptable conclusions to be drawn from any result after completion of the stated procedure. For example, a study to test the benefit from a certain binaural hearing aid might compare binaural and monaural scores from a group of hearing impaired subjects. Although the investigator might expect to find a significant difference between the two sets of scores, important conclusions could also be made if no difference appeared at all.

Occasionally when a thesis or dissertation is designed to support some favorite theory, the methodology may be structured only with significant results in mind, with no means to justify the opposite outcome. In such cases, which fortunately do not happen often, a failure to achieve significance could amount to failure of the entire project. An important question, therefore, that should be raised during the prospectus meeting is how well the proposal could also support unexpected or alternative results.

3. EVALUATION OF THE DATA

An initial statement of the probable statistics to be used will help to dictate the way in which the data are to be collected and grouped. By this means, the final arrangement of the data can be kept in mind throughout the study, as opposed to the frequent mistake of collecting the data first and then hoping that they will fit some kind of pattern later. The best data arrangement, as described in the section on statistical design, is to set up a proposed data analysis sheet in advance, so that the actual data collection will be essentially a matter of filling in the spaces under the appropriate group headings.

Criteria of measurement should be kept consistent throughout the study. Such things as alternate ways of scoring test results, or tabulating different kinds of parent reactions to the child may seem like good additions to the study, but the tactic of modifying techniques of data collection as the study progresses is likely to produce uneven groups of scores and weaken the subsequent statistical procedures.

Especially where the analysis of variance is to be used, the proposed data should be arranged tentatively according to the cells in the design in order to determine whether there are enough scores to fill out the pattern properly. Some types of data for the analysis of variance may also require the use of transformations, and this step should be anticipated well in advance of any computational procedure. The most common transformation is the substitution of arcsin values when the raw data are in the form of percentages.

4. AVAILABILITY OF SUBJECTS

A very common obstacle to the progress of a research project is the failure to find enough of a particular kind of subject needed for the data group. The prospectus meeting should be particularly critical toward studies that require a type of subject who is not readily available. These might include groups such as parents of stutterers, parents of cleft palate children, persons with sudden-onset hearing loss, or a narrowly-specified type of aphasic. Unless the population can be definitely assured in advance, the scope of the study should be modified to include subjects who are more available or to restructure the design so as to accommodate a smaller number of special subjects.

A factor that must be considered seriously in any study involving groups of seemingly plentiful school children, is the requirement by many school districts that special permission be obtained before the research involvement of any child in the school. The permission procedure varies widely from one district to the next, and may include anything from an informal agreement with the school principal to a formal review by the school board and signatures from all parents of the children to be involved. Because the school's objective is of course to provide an education for the child, the natural concern of the administration is to see that the child's schedule is not seriously interrupted or that the family's privacy is not invaded by the use of personal information. In addition, the method used to collect data should not give the parents any reason to believe that their child will be unfavorably classified or "set apart" by the experience. Finally, the regular classroom teacher may have justifiable concerns about intrusions into scheduled classroom activities through interruptions or absences caused by outside participation of some of the children. The details of permission for research in any school should, therefore, be clearly understood before plans are made to use school children in the project. However, in situation where the data can be collected without any additional testing or time involvement from the children, the study may simply be drawn informally from clinical information and therapy already in progress. This arrangement is usually appropriate for the full time clinician and, sometimes, for the student clinician with the help of the cooperating supervisor.

Regulations in the Use of Human Subjects

Since their publication in 1974, federal regulations concerning the use of human subjects for research purposes have had a major effect upon some research areas, notably in studies that involve electric shock conditioning, X-ray exposure, medication, or minor surgical techniques such as implantation of small electrode wires. Basically, the regulations, known as the National Research Act, Public Law 93–348, require the National Institutes of Health to be responsible for the rights of all human subjects who might be at risk through research funded by that agency. In actual practice, however, the regulations affect nearly all human research conducted anywhere under any circumstances. The only type of human research that is specifically exempt under the regulation is survey material, such as opinion polls, or question-naires relating to past experiences. Should the DHHS have reason to believe that any funded institution is conducting research that could put human subjects at risk, the agency is required to terminate any grants that are involved, and to take the incident into consideration in reviewing future grant proposals for that institution. Because most colleges and universities have some sort of federal funding, the far-reaching effects of the policy are obvious.

Looking beyond the stipulations of the law, however, it seems that profes-sional organizations and institutions in general have been increasingly con-cerned with research ethics and have been moving in the direction of stricter self-regulation. The American Psychological Association, for example, adopted a new set of ethics in 1973 that recommended the elimination of deceptive practices in research with human subjects. Some professional journals and convention programs have begun to recommend that studies that seem to involve some hazard or risk to human subjects should be accompanied by a statement indicating the precautions taken to insure their safety and welfare. Such assurances have now become routine on most campuses because one aspect of the federal regulations requires that an Institutional Review Board, consisting of at least five members must be established at each institution for the purpose of evaluating human subject research.

In planning research projects, three points should be kept in mind as a result of the National Research Act.

1. Some techniques reported in past literature may no longer be feasible. Perhaps the largest area to be effected is the use of X-ray photography on normal subjects. Clinical X-rays, however, may still be used in cases where they have always been part of the diagnostic procedure. Many other hazardous techniques, such as those involving certain drugs, may no longer be utilized even with the subject's written consent. Some techniques with minimal or questionable risk can be used only under special conditions.

2. The student should plan to fill out and submit the appropriate Human Subject Research forms if *any* human subjects are used in the proposed project, even though there may be quite obviously no risk involved. In most research situations, this brief extra step has simply become a routine part of the proposal.

3. The spirit of the Human Subject Research regulations implies that any research proposal should be reviewed before the project is actually begun. A late submission of the forms to the Institutional Review Board may halt the progress of the investigation until the proposal can be officially reviewed, and could cause an unfortunate delay in a tight time schedule.

5. ADEQUACY OF THE DATA SAMPLE

In planning the size of the data sample and the measures to be used, three areas of consideration should first be reviewed. These are the availability of subjects, measures per subject, and type and quantity of measures needed for valid test results.

The first point is related to the earlier discussion on the availability of special types of subjects. For example, it would be unrealistic in most situations to base a study upon the likelihood that 100 cases of laryngectomy, aphasia, or shuttering would be currently available. Many investigations of specialized disorders are based upon ten or less subjects. For a general rule, as the disorder is more narrowly defined, fewer subjects will be found who fit exactly into the category. In a study to evaluate the speech from an innovative reed-fistula surgical procedure in laryngectomees, only four subjects were used (Weinberg *et al.*, 1978). Because the total population for this type of speaker is extremely small, a test sample of four is as large as one could realistically expect.

The second point relates to the amount (or depth) of testing to be conducted on each subject. In the speech and hearing science area, in which the research is likely to involve basic psychophysical methods, a large sample of data might be gleaned from a very small number of subjects, or even a single subject. A rather exhaustive study on the dynamics of normal respiration was conducted from data on only three subjects (Hixon, *et al.*, 1976). Survey studies, however, require less data per subject, but derive their reliability from much larger populations, as shown in a categorization of the speech of Parkinson patients (Logemann *et al.*, 1978) in which 200 subjects were included.

Particularly where a very small number of normal subjects are used, however, it is assumed that the subjects have been carefully chosen, so as to eliminate the possible influence of some unique individual characteristics. In the speech science area, this usually means that the subjects are entirely free from all speech and hearing anomalies, and are representative of the population in general.

The final, and perhaps the most important consideration in sample size, is the requirement of the amount of data necessary for the proposed statistical computation. Most statistics are designed for use with a certain optimum number of subjects. An analysis of variance, for instance, can easily handle large samples, but it is often used with 10 to 15 subjects per experimental group, and with no fewer than five scores per cell. Statistics based upon normal distribution, such as the t-test or the r coefficient of correlation should include enough scores to display a reasonably normal distribution. Nonparametric statistics, on the other hand, are intended for smaller samples, in which the number of scores would usually not go beyond 30.

A general layout of the proposed data will relieve much of the confusion in estimating whether the groups of numbers in the computation are going to be sufficient to yield realistic means or averages in each set of measures. For example, it would be unrealistic to estimate a mean on the basis of only two or three measures; where the scores show wide variability, a greater number, such as 10, 20 or 30 may be necessary in order to find a good representative average for the sample.

From the preceding discussion, it becomes apparent that the investigator's insight into the subject matter will play some role into the estimate of appropriate sample size and concommitant statistical preference. For instance, the speech reception threshold from five young adults with normal ears should be expected to yield a highly predictable mean, and a larger sample would be unlikely to improve the accuracy of the estimate. On the other hand, speech reception thresholds from five aphasics might show extreme variability, so as to give an average score that would not really represent the group's performance.

Although a computational approach to the estimate of sample size is usually not superior to an educated guess, some readers may wish to use a method described by Winer (Winer, 1971, p. 104), in which an equation may be set up to show the relationship among the number of treatments, the number of scores per treatment, and the desired level of statistical significance. The equation is structured for use with the analysis of variance. However, as Winer points out, the estimate of population variance to be used in the formula depends upon the best guess from the investigator.

6. AVAILABILITY OF EQUIPMENT

An additional potential problem to the collection of data is the availability and reliability of specialized equipment to be used in the study. Although some standard equipment is set up for use on a continuous basis, as in hearing test equipment, many types of apparatus require considerable adjustment before performance becomes reliable. It is, therefore, imperative to set up the equipment and to run a few subjects before the final plan of investigation is arranged. In most instances, the use of lab equipment implies also the reservation of enough space in which to set up a working arrangement for running subjects.

As a rule of thumb, the more units of equipment to be used, the greater is the likelihood of unexpected equipment failure. This generalization may be applied also to the number of people who are currently using the same apparatus. The types of equipment failure are literally unlimited, but some of the more common problems included:

Background hum, which is usually 60 Hz, and originates mostly from other electrical devices being used in the same room or building. Fluorescent lights, generators, electric motors, and X-ray machines are common sources of hums or buzzes. Some of the offending sources, such as certain lights, can be turned off. Most other electrical noise can be "drained off" if new ground lines are installed in the room or if shielded wire is used. For extremely sensitive equipment, such as electromyograph or brain wave recorders, the entire room may have to be enclosed with well grounded copper screening.

Small units of equipment are sometimes battery-powered, which makes them entirely free from hum and electrical line noises. At the present time, however, battery power is not widely used in experimental work, mainly because some units are too large for this type of power, and precise equipment tends to run more uniformly and to last longer if it is simply plugged in and left on rather than turned on and off for each period of use.

Loss of signal strength is usually from a mismatch of impedance in the hook-up between two pieces of equipment. *Impedance* refers to the total load of electrical resistance under which the unit is designed to operate. For instance, most headphones are low impedance units, but a few are designed with high impedance. To avoid impedance mismatch, it is helpful to mark the signal input connections on electrical equipment as to their specified impedance ratings in ohms. If both pieces of equipment function at similar ohms (within 10% of each rating), the signal will not be weakened. Other causes of weak signal strength include improper setting of the equipment adjustments and the use of patch cords and electrical extension lines that are too long and tend to add resistance in the line.

Intermittant loss of signal can be caused by a heavy use of electical power at certain hours of the day. This results in a temporary drop of voltage that may be enough to weaken or eliminate the output from some units for a period of time. To prevent this disturbance, some labs have a voltage regulator installed in the main power line, which helps to maintain an even flow of electricity to the equipment. Other causes for intermittant loss of signal may be weak electrical parts that overheat or possibly, too much apparatus plugged into the same line at certain times.

Interjection of a local radio station signal occurs mainly when the station is within a mile or two of the experimental equipment. It is caused by having too many long wires running between the electronic components, and also by the settings of some amplifier and filter circuits, which may inadvertently tune in to the radio frequency. It is both annoying and humorous to hear music and weather reports coming through the playback monitor at a time when some delicate speech signal or muscle signal is being recorded. In one bizarre instance, an investigator was astounded to hear Christmas carols coming from the surface electrodes of a cat's brain! In most cases, a more efficient hook-up of the apparatus will solve the problem, but in extreme situations, a grounded copper screen enclosure may be the only solution.

As one might imagine, the process of "debugging" a set of assembled apparatus is frustrating and tedious, and the best approach is to leave the equipment essentially untouched except for the actual experiment, once the troubleshooting procedure has been successful.

7. TIME PERIOD ALLOTTED FOR THE STUDY

Although many theses and dissertations are completed after the student finishes all other requirements and leaves campus, the risk of failure to complete the study becomes greater with each semester away from the university. It is, therefore, of critical importance to complete all of the data collection and all or most of the computation and writing while the student is still in residence. From the standpoint of the student, two relatively common causes of delay should be resolved in advance. These are the availability of the thesis advisor and clear criteria to determine completion of the work.

Responsibilities or tentative future commitments that will take the advisor away from campus for frequent or extended periods present a serious obstacle that is not uncommon to the delay of theses and dissertations. Major decisions in the progress of the study should normally be cleared with the advisor as the situation arises. These include unexpected modifications in the number or type of subjects to be used, alternative procedures due to equipment failure, or the addition of extra steps in data processing, all of which can develop with annoying predictability in spite of the most careful planning. Finally, the approval of the written manuscript must be granted by the advisor before the departmental and university acceptance of the finished work. When the advisor is unavailable at these crucial times, the department may be forced to make substitute arrangements, placing the project into a situation of uncertain status, in which the previous agreements must be reviewed. Although it is a faculty committee that makes the final decision on the acceptance of the student's research project, the advisor's position is weighed very heavily in these matters. In nearly all cases of failure in thesis or dissertation orals, the problem may be traced to the student's failure or inability to work closely with the advisor.

The second aspect of involvement for the student to consider is the criterion for determining when the study is completed, as indicated by the written procedure and the formal questions to be answered by the study. In most cases, the written prospectus represents a tentative approval of the scope of the study on the part of the faculty advisory committee. Failure to have a rather firm agreement as to the projected outcome of the study might lead to a tendency to add additional questions to the study or to expand the area of the topic. This tendency is the natural result of scientific curiosity and may develop without awareness, until the student finds that the study has somehow gradually been expanded into a much larger endeavor than was first undertaken. In extreme instances of this situation, neither the student nor his advisors have maintained a clear criterion for concluding the project, and the work seems to drift along past the deadlines without a well-defined goal.

Although procrastination plays at least a minor role in nearly all research projects, there are some aspects of delay that can be reduced through awareness and advanced planning. Some projects, for instance, are naively conceived to provide the entire conclusive answer for a major research area. The scope of such ambitious plans is usually not realistic for the time frame of graduate study; the law which applies to advanced planning is that *research is never simpler than planned—it is always more complicated.* Related to this general situation, particularly with a doctoral dissertation, is a tendency to be overly perfectionistic. Perfection to some extent is of course built in to the rigor of a thorough investigation, but a preoccupation with trivia adds nothing but time to the study.

In extreme examples, the student's commitment to his research project may become almost a way of life, in which new facets are continually added to the study, with no apparent aim toward a firm date of termination. Completion of the project within the given time period must be viewed as an important part of the training experience, with responsibility shared by the student and the advisor. Because deadlines nearly always apply to funded research or to academic time allotments for sponsored projects, the ability to pace the project properly to the expected completion date should be developed as part of the total research learning experience.

CHAPTER 5   **Research Concepts and Terminology**

As the research project develops, various areas of unfamiliar concepts and terminology are encountered at each stage. Research like most other disciplines, has a vocabulary of its own, and a better comprehension of the terminology increases the awareness of context and perspective of the project as a whole. Included in the list that follows are some of the more common research terms, principally those which supply helpful background for choices and decisions which will need to be made as the student's project develops.

BASIC AND APPLIED RESEARCH

As mentioned in an earlier section, all research may be divided into basic research or applied research. In the field of communication disorders, clinical research is primarily applied research, and speech and hearing science falls mostly into the category of basic research. Some examples will, of course, fall under both headings, and from a philosophical standpoint, this type may make the most significant contribution to the field. In their purest forms, however, basic research is intended only to decipher the laws of nature and applied research is designed only to answer a practical question. From time to time, we read the remarks of Nobel scientists and other dedicated researchers who deplore the lack of basic research in progress, pointing out that it is a kind of natural resource that must be replenished and maintained up-to-date in order to supply the basis of a growing technology. In contrast to the immediate benefits from applied research, the results of basic research are intended for storage, to accumulate in the archives until someone can put them together to make a new scientific advancement. At the moment, the talking computer (and similarly, the talking speech aid for nonverbal persons) is perhaps the best example of a technical advancement which has been made possible through years of basic research dealing with vowel formants, phoneme transitions, and similar studies in the acoustic science of speech. Another application that will mark the assemblage of years of basic research might be the implanted hearing aid, which is now still in the early experimental stage.

Because applied research is clearly easier for most legislators to understand and appreciate, federal sponsorhsip of research endeavor tends for the most part to lean toward solutions to problems that confront our society or impede our technology. The general public itself, is perhaps even more critical of basic research, as being a waste of time because the results seem to serve no immediate purpose. Ideally, of course, each type of research supports the other. Applied research cannot advance without basic information, and basic research becomes a sterile exercise if it is never needed by an advancing technical field.

RETROSPECTIVE (EX POST FACTO) STUDIES AND EXPERIMENTAL STUDIES

The Latin term *ex post facto* indicates that the research was conducted "after the fact", or after the event has already occurred. Similarly, *retrospective* denotes that the researcher is looking back at something that has happened at an earlier time. This designation is given to research in which the condition to be studied is already present and the experimenter has no control over it. Thus, if the condition to be studied is stuttering or hearing loss, the experimenter must accept the condition as it is and assume that this is the only factor being observed. This is a very weak assumption in some cases because the experimental subjects may have had other experiences which would influence the outcome of the study as much as the disorder itself. For example, a deaf person may have not only a lack of hearing, but a lack of education as well. The main point is that the experimenter had no control over the circumstances relating to the subject's condition whereas, in a strictly experimental study, the experimenter would start with a group of randomly chosen subjects and assign them equally to each condition. The fact that individuals in real life are not assigned to become stutterers, articulation cases, or other clinical populations is considered—technically at least— to be a weakness in this type of study. Conversely, the purely laboratory study in which all variables can be meticulously controlled is sometimes criticized because it does not deal with natural events as they actually occur in real life situations.

Statistically, the power of the *ex post facto* study is slightly weakened because an entirely pure sample of a certain disorder cannot be obtained; there is always an uncontrolled aspect in the selection process. One way to overcome this weakness is to increase the size of the sample so as to minimize the effect of atypical cases which might have been included. With many types of communicative disorders, however, larger samples are not available. Young (1976) recommends that a statistical procedure called *regression analysis* be used in retrospective research, in which the effect of the clinical group classification might be used to isolate the clinical condition from other unwanted factors that could be influencing the result. Regression analysis, which is a computerized method, has the advantage of being able to evaluate an almost unlimited number of factors at the same time, and to assess the degree of influence that each has upon the final outcome.

NORMAL DISTRIBUTION AND NONPARAMETRIC DISTRIBUTION

Normal distribution of statistical data means that the scores tend to fall into a bell-shaped curve, with the majority of scores clustering around the middle of the range. The term *normal* implies that most groups of scores in nature seem to have this pattern. The concept is easily illustrated in body weights, in which most people are of "medium" weight, with some people weighing more than average, and about an equal number weighing less than average. Many of the most common statistics are designed to be used with normally distributed data. These include the t-tests, the F, and the Pearson r. Normal distribution statistics make the assumption that the scores are scattered evenly around the mean, and if the data do not take this standard form, the result could be invalid.

Particularly with the sudden popularity of the analysis of variance in the mid-50s, great emphasis was placed upon meeting the criterion of normal distribution, or at least consistency among the group distributions, which is called *homogeneity of variance*. It seemed necessary, therefore, to check all groups for the proper variance by a technique called *Bartlet's Test*, before the main statistical analysis could be run. More recently, however, the *robust* nature of most statistical formulas is better understood, which means that the assumptions that underlie most statistics can be violated slightly without disturbing their accuracy. If, however, the data are clearly not in a normal distribution, a nonparametric statistic should be used.

A number of empirical obervations can be used to check for normal distribution when the variance of the data is uncertain.

1. The mean and the median should be nearly identical. In other words, the average should fall in the middle of the scores.
2. The greater number of scores should cluster around the middle of the distribution, with no clustering at the high or the low end of the range.
3. In most random samples normal distribution can be assumed if the sample size exceeds 30 scores.

Nonparametric distributions may take several forms. One of the most common is the rank order data arrangement, in which all the test items—such as hearing aids, voice samples, cleft palates, etc.—are simply arranged in numerical order from highest to lowest according to some characteristic. This type of data has no clustering and no central tendency. Other examples of nonparametric distributions include data in which most of the scores cluster at either or both ends of the range instead of the middle, or where the sample is so small that no central tendency appears. In the cases, the data must be converted into ranks or binomial data before statistics can be applied. A borderline area of nonparametric distribution is composed of data that were derived from a seven-point scale or similar rating technique. Although the data are based on a type of ranked scores, the group may be found to have normal distribution. Conservatively, the situation might call for a nonparametric statistic although normal distribution statistics have also been used effectively, particularly with larger samples.

It is not unusual for the student to think that a nonparametric treatment is somehow inferior, perhaps because those statistics are generally easier to compute and may seem, therefore, to be at a more elementary level. If anything, a review of journal articles would probably lead to the opposite conclusion, and the ability to select the most appropriate nonparametric method requires good statistical insight and competence. Although normal distribution statistics are slightly more sensitive to significant differences, a properly used nonparametric treatment is superior to an incorrectly used normal distribution statistic.

HYPOTHESIS

In order to determine whether or not the investigation answers the question that has been proposed, the topic is worded in the form of a statement, which may either be supported or rejected by the results of the analysis. It should be obvious that the statement must be succinctly worded, because a vague hypothesis will not result in a definite conclusion. In most studies, as discussed in more detail in a later section, there are actually two hypotheses: a formal and an informal statement. The formal hypothesis is worded in the terms of "no difference" or "no relationship", and should include the criterion measurements for deciding whether or not to reject the hypothesis: "There is no difference in hearing performance for the two types of hearing aids, as measured by discrimination test scores."Clearly, a significant difference in scores for the two types of hearing aids will mean that the hypothesis may be rejected. The formal hypothesis, being worded negatively, is called a *null hypothesis*. Because this is the more conservative approach to natural phenomena, it states that most events are coincidence or chance happenings unless shown to be otherwise.

The other type of hypothesis is the informal statement or question, called the *working hypothesis*. This is worded in the way the investigator is actually thinking of his project, such as, "Is there a difference between the speech rates of stutterers and nonstutterers?" Either the null hypothesis or the working hypothesis may be used in the published report of the investigation, but the mathematical theory behind the statistics is based on the acceptance or rejection of the null hypothesis.

RELIABILITY

A fundamental question about any research study is, "If the study were done again, would the result be the same?" This refers to the reliability of the study. Reliability is influenced by the *size* of the sample, the *control* of the variables, and the *precision* of the measurements. Within the study itself, however, judges are often used to make some qualitative measurement, such as the relative intelligibility of speech samples, voice quality, or progress in speech therapy. When this method is used, it is advisable to find how well the judges agree with each other, or how much a judge will agree with himself if the trials are repeated. Judges' agreement with each other is called *interjudge* reliability, and agreement with themselves is called *intrajudge* reliability.

Several tests are used to indicate the degree of reliability of a study. The most frequent methods are expressed as *percentage* of agreement, *correlations* between measures, and *standard error* of the mean for each measure. For good reliability, judges should agree on at least 90% of their judgments. Correlations between judges' ratings are usually reported with an r of at least .88 or better. The standard error in certain measurements is reported as an indication of reliability for repeated measurements of the same items. In X-ray measures, for example, the standard error is often reported as .5 millimeters. This means that if the X-ray pictures were measured by someone else, the new average measures will probably be within .5 millimeters of the original ones.

SIGNIFICANCE, LEVEL OF CONFIDENCE, AND PROBABILITY

Upon the completion of nearly any statistical treatment, the result is presented in terms of its significance, expressed as the level of confidence. This concept is explained in statistical texts by illustrating the familiar bell-shaped curve and referring to the narrow end segment at the tail of the curve to indicate how small the possibility is for a statistical error. The confidence level of the result is the possibility of having made an error, or in other words, how confident we are that we have not made an error. So, the .05 level of confidence means that there are five chances out of 100 that the result could be wrong. The .01 level of confidence means that there is only one chance in 100 of having arrived at a false statistical result. In a general sense probability, significance, and level of confidence all refer to essentially the same thing, that is, how sure we can be of our result.

As a simplified rule of thumb, if the investigation is to show that a significant difference exists, we prefer to use a level of confidence that is less than .01. If the study is to conclude that a significant difference does *not* exist, it is usually shown by a level of confidence which exceeds .05. This means that we usually wish to be 99% sure that a significant difference exists, and if we are not at least 95% confident of a difference, we prefer to say that there is no real difference at all.

We occasionally hear the argument that research never actually *proves* anything; it only supports or does not support a hypothesis. This is simply a semantic consideration of the word *prove*, based upon the use of probability. Theoretically, at least, even if our result is significant at the .001 level, we have still left open the thousand-to-one possibility that the conclusion could be false. Strictly speaking, to prove something implies there is no possible chance for error—a condition that theoretically does not exist in statistics.

TYPES OF DATA SCALES

Although the classification of data obtained by various measuring techniques may appear at first to be merely an academic detail, it is quite important and very practical to be aware of the types of statistical treatment that must be used with each class of data.

Interval Scale

This is the scale that we use in everyday counting and simple arithmetic. The main feature of this scale is that there is equal distance between units; that is, the distance between three and four is the same as the distance between 10 and 11. This scale is the most useful of the data systems from a statistical standpoint because it contains the most information and lends itself well to regular normal distribution techniques. For optimal use, the range of these data should not be restricted, and with each sample, other criteria for normal distribution (i.e., the bulk of the scores should cluster around the center, etc.) should also be incorporated for maximum statistical advantage. The interval scale, especially when used in units of one is very sensitive to small differences and, therefore, tends to avoid tied scores. Generally speaking, tied scores are not particularly helpful in statistical computation, and they can sometimes be eliminated by using more precision and a smaller type of unit in the raw measurements.

In theory, when there is no limit to the size of the measuring unit or the precision that can be used, the measures are called *continuous data*. This is one form of the interval scale. It implies that any unit used for this particular measurement provides just an estimate of the actual value. If we were to say that someone's vocal cords are one inch long, it is just an estimate of their actual length; they could be 27 millimeters long, or 111 microns long, depending upon which unit one chooses to use and how much precision can realistically be achieved. When the measures cannot be broken into smaller units, however, they represent *discrete data*, which are usually in the form of objects or events to be counted. These could be the number of hair cells, correct responses, voice cases, hearing aids, stuttering blocks, or children. Although it may be possible to have half of a hair cell, half of a hearing aid, or even half a person, anything less than the whole is not a real unit, and for this reason, they are termed discrete units. Other measures that are customarily treated as discrete data are tests of I.Q., articulation scores, hearing discrimination, and language skills. From a practical standpoint, the research areas of speech, language, and hearing usually deal with measures that are rounded off into whole units, because most concepts in behavioral sciences are not by nature well-suited to hairline precision.

When a set of inteval data falls into an apparently normal distribution, as described earlier, the statistical treatments usually include the t-tests, the F-test analysis of variance, and the Pearson coefficient of correlation. When the interval data fall into some form of nonnormal distribution, such as being bimodal, skewed, or completely flat, the interval scores may be transformed into rank order (the ordinal scale) for use with nonparametric statistics.

Ordinal Scale: Rank Order

When comparative characteristics are lined up in rank order, the arrangement is referred to as ranked data, which uses the ordinal scale. Use of this type of measure implies that the characteristic being measured does not lend itself to interval data, or that the interval data were not normally distributed. An excellent example of the appropriate use of ordinal data is in the rank order of brain specimens for a study concerning relative deterioration in aphasia (Sklar, 1963). Because a part of the study was to determine how each brain compared to the rest of the group, there were no numbers that could be used to give a real "score" to each brain, and the rank order scale was used. Further, ordinal data do not imply that there are equal units between numbers, so that number one may be considerably better or only slightly better than number two.

Even though normal distribution is not assumed in this scale, ordinal data make a very good substitute for interval data, and the statistics are about 95% as effective in detecting similarities and differences as those used with normal distribution. Rank order techniques include the major nonparametric statistics, such as the Mann-Whitney U, the Wilcoxon T, and the two nonparametric versions of the analysis of variance—the Friedman test and the Kruskal-Wallis H. For correlation, the Spearman rho is used. Most of the statistics designed for ordinal data will yield basically the same result as interval data in the majority of cases, as discussed by Siegal (1956). The only serious shortcoming in ordinal data is that they cannot be used in the types of analysis of variance that test for interactions among factors.

Nominal Data

As the term implies, nominal data involve simply assigning a name or category to each item. For example, the resulting test score might be designated "pass" or "fail." When only two categories of this nature are used, the data are called *binomial*. Other typical examples of binomial data are yes-no, plus-minus, or improved-not improved.

In other instances, nominal data may be in the form of tallies under several different headings, as in survey studies where children are classified according to Latino, Caucasian, or Black, or according to types of disorders, such as articulation, voice, or fluency. In survey studies, the results are usually reported as the number or percentage of individuals found in each of the nominal categories. Unlike the preceding data scales, nominal data do not imply that any of the categories represents a higher or lower value or rank than the others. Even when a 1-0 classification is used, the category of 0 has as much weight as the category of 1.

The most frequently used statistic with nominal data is the chi square. With simple two-group comparisons, particularly when the scores are plus-minus, the sign test is used.

DEPENDENT AND INDEPENDENT VARIABLES

Which factor is being changed as a result of the other? The factor that is being changed is the *dependent variable*, and the factor that remains controlled is the *independent variable*. In a test of auditory discrimination, the investigator may obtain scores for a group of subjects with and without hearing aids. The variable being controlled is the presence or absence of the hearing aid; this is the independent variable, and is arranged in advance by the investigator. The variable that is influenced by whether or not a hearing aid is being worn is the discrimination test score; this is the dependent variable. Typically, independent variables in this field include age, sex, type of therapy, type of hearing loss, or race. Dependent variables usually are some kind of performance measures, such as test scores, hearing thresholds, judges' evaluations, or questionnaire responses.

Although this seems to be a relatively elementary concept, the role of each variable is sometimes lost as the student constructs the procedure and results sections of the project, and a clear designation of which variables are dependent and independent helps to outline the outcome with less confusion. In more complicated studies, however, the author may actually point out the dependent and independent variables to simplify the analysis for the reader:

"Figure 3 shows the results of this analysis, the dependent variable being the proportion of stutterers at each of the combined levels of independent variables."

(Griggs and Still, 1979, p. 576)

VALIDITY

How well does the research answer the question being studies? In the thesis or dissertation, the question of validity should be raised at the prospectus meeting and again at the oral defense of the study. Two areas of validity must be considered: internal validity and external validity.

Internal Validity

Internal validity refers mostly to the control of experimental variables and elimination of extraneous factors that might bias the result. Extraneous factors include sex differences, age, subject fatigue, subject motivation, hall noise, distractions, learning effects between tests, socioeconomic level, and I.Q. It is customary to counterbalance or match the various groups of subjects so as to eliminate the influence of all possible factors except the ones being investigated. When all spurious factors are eliminated or neutralized, and the only factors left in the experiment are the clearly defined independent and dependent variables, the experimental design is considered to have high internal validity. This is often referred to as a "clean" experiment, indicating that there are no contaminating influences. Because clinical research must deal with conditions, disorders, and people as they exist in real life, it is impossible to have absolute control over all possible variables, and clinical studies are, therefore, considered to have somewhat lower internal validity than laboratory studies.

External Validity

External validity means how well the study relates to the real world. Factors that influence external validity include sample size, selection of subjects, use of control groups, and interpretation of the results. Clinical studies that are based upon very small samples, one-subject studies, and laboratory studies that do not allow for real life considerations, tend to lack external validity. A hearing aid, for example, which is researched only under strict laboratory conditions may be practically useless in the real life environment of traffic noise, office noise, or loud speech.

A PRIORI AND A POSTERIORI JUDGMENTS

A priori refers to conclusions or judgments drawn before the statistical analysis, and *a posteriori* refers to conclusions drawn after the primary statistical computation is made.

Some of the most common a priori judgments include the selection of sample size, choice of the proper individual for one-subject studies, or determination of the most realistic level of confidence. Most a priori judgments depend upon the investigator's familiarity with the research population or with models of previous studies on the topic. For example, where subjects are well known to be homogeneous, as in the hearing of normal young adults, an a priori estimate of sample size might include only five subjects. A more diverse type of data, such as job attitudes of school speech clinicians should probably sample at least 50 people for an estimate, and might well require 100 or 200 respondents in order to make a representative survey.

In a more formal way, a priori judgment refers to a statistical procedure called *planned comparisons*, in which a t-test or similar comparison is made before computation of the analysis of variance. By this treatment method, the most important area can be compared first, and the F-test is then used as a follow-up sort of screening test to check for additional comparisons that could also be of interest.

A posteriori comparisons are typically made after the determination of a significant F-test over one or more factors in the analysis of variance. The analysis of variance in this case is analogous to a large net that is dragged through the groups of data to see whether or not any significant differences appear. If the net should come up empty, there is no need to examine the data any further. However, if one or more significant F-test results appear, the investigator may decide either that the research question has already been satisfactorily answered, or else that it is now necessary to find in greater detail exactly which groups differ from each other. Further testing after a significant F-test is called a posteriori testing or *post hoc* analysis. By this method, the a posteriori testing is used to point out the more important details of the results. Tests for post hoc analysis include the Tukey, Newman-Keuls, Scheffe, and sometimes the t-test.

TYPE I AND TYPE II STATISTICAL ERRORS

In any statistical treatment, there is room for error. The chance for error in each result is displayed along with the value of the result, such as $F = 12.85, p. < .01$. In this example, the analysis of variance was significant, with only one chance in 100 (.01) that the result is erroneous. This assumes that the computation itself is accurate, and refers only to how certain we are that the result did not come about by accident. If a significant result does occur by accident, it is called a Type I error. Therefore, a Type I error can be avoided by using the lowest possible probability level.

In the simplest terms, the Type I error means that a significant result appeared statistically, when in fact it was not really there. Generally speaking, the chance of committing a Type I error is increased if the sample is too small, if some irregular scores are discarded, or if the probability level is too liberal.

Type II errors are less frequently made, and are inclined to occur when the variability of a sample is so great that the potentially significant result is obscured, or that the use of a less sensitive statistic did not distinguish the subtle differences. A Type II error is, therefore, the opposite of the Type I, in that a significant result was actually present in the experiment, but the investigator did not use methods or treatments sensitive enough to reveal it.

In theory, the Type I and Type II errors are considered equally to be avoided, but in practice, the Type I error could have the poorer connotation, in that the investigator may seem too eager to present results that are not well founded.

A matter somewhat analogous to the Type I and Type II errors are the interpretations that are customarily drawn from the results and presented in the Conclusion section at the end of the report. In this section, the investigator may be guilty of deriving either too much or too little from the statistical results. At times, too much is made of "nonsignificant trends" or of comparisons that "just miss significance." In other instances, the over-cautious researcher may raise so many points of contention that the reader cannot appreciate the study's legitimate contribution, and the fact that significant results were actually found.

ONE-TAILED AND TWO-TAILED TESTS

With any statistical comparison of two groups, the investigator must decide on an a priori basis whether one group can definitely be assumed to have slightly higher scores than the other. In comparing language scores, for example, between a group of 5-year-olds and a group of 6-year-olds, we would assume in advance that the 6-year-olds will score slightly higher; our research question is whether or not this difference is actually significant. In this type of situation, the result should be checked on the statistical probability tables under the heading of a *one-tailed test*. This means that the two groups may differ only in one direction; the older children might score higher or might score the same as the younger children, but they will not score lower than the younger group. If a marginally significant difference exists between the two groups, there is a slight advantage to be gained in the level of confidence by accepting a one-tailed instead of a two-tailed test, because the level of confidence (i.e., chance for error) is only half as great in the one-tailed test. To illustrate, if we had obtained a t-test result of 1.85 with 20 degrees of freedom, a one-tailed test would be significant at better than the .05 level of confidence ($p. < .05$). The same result in a two-tailed test would exceed .05 ($p. > .05$), which would usually be considered nonsignificant.

The terms *one-tailed* and *two-tailed* tests refer to the outline of the normal distribution curves for the two groups of data being compared. The one-tailed test implies that the two groups can overlap only at one end of the curve, that is at one "tail" of the normal curve. The two-tailed test implies that the two groups can differ in either direction or, in other words, at two tails of the curve. Most comparisons are two-tailed tests, because higher scores for one of the groups cannot usually be assumed in advance. As a rule of thumb, if there is some question of which approach to use, the two-tailed test is the better choice, leading to a more conservative result.

CHAPTER 6

The Use of Computers and Calculators in Research

The mystique of the computer as an instrument for research sometimes connotes the idea that the computer does all the work by itself and takes the place of the human in some respects. In some television shows, the computer is displayed as having a human speaking voice and all the stored knowledge of several encyclopedias. Such a computer could easily display the wiring diagrams of all makes of audiometers, retrieve clinical documents, print out the abstracts of any group of research articles or perhaps tell us which statistic to use for a given set of data. All of these functions are in fact within the realm of reality, except for one very time-consuming prerequisite: someone must first sit for hours or weeks at the computer and make up the computer programs, type in all of the encyclopedic material, abstracts, and statistical treatments, and store everything on the computer's tapes, cassettes, or punch cards. This, as one could well imagine, is a highly limiting feature of computer use, and often leaves us with the alternative of simply looking up the material or doing computations with a hand calculator rather than to bother with the cumbersome nature of the computer. The second restricting feature of the computer might be termed its mindless compulsivity. If, for example, we were to omit an item such as a space, comma, or semicolon in the program for a three factor analysis involving 100 subjects, the computer might quit in the first stages of the program, may give meaningless results, or could proceed to print out ten pages of data that were not intended. It is relatively rare for the average computer user to get the right answer on the first try with a new computer program. In summary, we can easily see that although the computer is extremely fast, extremely accurate, tireless (although it does need regular service and repair), and capable of very large and complicated projects, it requires a great deal of time and patience on the part of the user.

THE HAND CALCULATOR

At the bottom of the hierarchy in the family of electronic data control technology is the inexpensive hand calculator. The cost of the cheaper models puts them in the category of throw-away materials, along with the plastic wrist watch, and the small pocket radio. Considering the rather negligible investment involved, there is little need for a consumer report; one small calculator works about as well as the next. However, the statistician is well-advised to select a calculator which—at the very least—includes the square root function.

47

At the next level of hand calculators are those that include added functions for specialized use. These are often labeled "the statistician", or "the scientific calculator." For a few extra dollars, these models typically include two or three additional functions that are very useful in statistics, along with several other functions that may never be used at all. Among the most helpful are the automatic summation, the mean, and the standard deviation. These save a number of extra steps in almost all statistical computations. A less-used but nonetheless valuable feature is the arcsin trigonometric function, which is used to transform percentage data before computing the analysis of variance. At a still more advanced level, some of the more expensive hand calculators have a function called "sums of squares." This is not to be confused with sums of squares found in the results of the analysis of variance, but indicates merely that each data value is squared, and that all the squared values are then added up. This is a preliminary step to many statistical computations.

PROGRAMMABLE HAND CALCULATORS

Programmable hand calculators are about the same size as the common drug store variety of hand calculator, but their cost of several hundred dollars and their computer-like capability puts them into an entirely more advanced classification. Unfortunately, most programmable hand calculators do not live up to expectations. The most obvious shortcoming is that whenever most calculators are turned off, the program is lost. This means that unless one plans to do at least three or four t-tests in a row, there is little time to be gained by setting up the program, as opposed to working the problem by hand from a book example. Fortunately, some newer models can retain the program even in the "off" mode. The second shortcoming is in the limited storage capacity of this type of unit, which confines most of them to fairly simple statistical formulas. A few programmable calculators have a storage capacity on small strips of magnetic tape, so that the program can be saved for future use. However, the limited capacity in the number of steps that can be stored is highly restricting, and this shortcoming should be weighed heavily against the expense involved. A very few programmable calculators also have built-in programs for several of the most-used statistics, such as the t-test and the Pearson r. This valuable feature is usually used more than the programmable capacity.

THE MICROCOMPUTER

Available at a remarkably low price is the microcomputer, or "home computer", which is available at electronics centers and department stores and looks somewhat like a typewriter with a small TV screen mounted on top. The advertising for these units would lead us to believe that a junior high school student would sit at the set to perform his or her homework, the housewife would use it for storage of cooking recipes, and that we would use it for quick and efficient balancing of the family checkbook, not to mention statistical computation. Although all these functions are possible, none are very realistic for the average person at the present time. The main bottleneck for use of the microcomputer is the lack of software. *Software* refers to programs already made up to be available commercially on cassettes. Although the future for these "canned programs" is extremely promising they are not yet available in sufficient variety to serve many purposes. Most of the currently available programs consist of games, quizzes, and similar novelties, although more practical materials are gradually appearing on the market. In addition, the use of cassette tapes as the principle method of program and data storage is time-consuming, cumbersome, and sometimes unreliable. For instance, if we were to store the clinical data from 100 subjects on a single cassette, it might be necessary to wait while the tape played through the entire cassette before the desired subject's record were found and the information displayed on the screen. In contrast to the rather rugged sound recording capability of cassette recorders, the delicate nature of computer code makes it imperative that the tape recording heads be kept clean and in excellent working condition if the programs or data are to be retrieved. Materials that were not recorded at good signal strength fade from the cassette in a few days and, therefore, cannot be recalled from the memory. The commercially available programs on cassette, however, are very reliable. A print-out attachment is also available, as well as substantial differences in the program capacity (the number of *bytes*) among various models. The serious user will wish to obtain the model with the larger capacity. These additions may increase the cost of the unit considerably. As more software becomes available, these units will undoubtedly enjoy great popularity, and may eliminate the need for computer terminals in many research programs, because they can perform all but the most complicated statistical functions.

MINICOMPUTERS

Intermediate between the microcomputer and the full sized computer is the minicomputer, which is roughly the size of a file cabinet. Its primary field of service is in business corporations that have the need to link a number of branch offices. These computers are designed to function in linked systems in which current information and reports are constantly being updated and summarized. COBAL and BASIC are their most common languages. Working in combination, their total capacity and capability is on par with that of the full sized computer. Being of intermediate size, their function and expense is beyond the scope of individuals or small research programs, which would be better served by a terminal from a full sized computer.

FULL SIZED COMPUTERS

The full sized computer, available for research purposes at most universities, offers maximum capability in data analysis and organization, but sacrifices simplicity of programming as it gains in versatility. Unless one is to become a consistent computer user, the expertise of programming is a full discipline in itself, and one in which the occasional user easily becomes lost. This is not to suggest, however, that the aspiring researcher should avoid learning the fundamentals of programming; a certain basic familiarity with computer language is necessary in order to interact on common ground with a professional programmer. In particular, the ability to find and correct minor errors in spacing, spelling, or punctuation that would abort the program or produce erroneous results is an invaluable asset to the computer user. Workshops and short courses are helpful for learning the techniques of modifying or "debugging" computer programs. There is no substitute for hands-on learning by the process of running one's own program. The aspiring computer user is, therefore, encouraged to run a few practice programs and to experiment with making modifications in order to gain personal experience as an adjunct to learning through lectures and readings in the subject.

Rather than attempting to be a comprehensive computer programmer, those who plan to use the computer on an occasional basis for research purposes usually concentrate on developing a few specific programs that will serve their needs and increase in familiarity through frequent use. For example, in addition to the common t-tests and Pearson r, computer programs for a three-factor analysis of variance with repeated measures, and a stepwise multiple regression may serve the statistical needs for a wide variety of investigations. Simpler statistics, including the chi square and nonparametric techniques, as well as the t and r may also be performed on the computer, but unless computer access is extremely convenient these can usually be conducted more readily on the hand calculator. Some centers prefer that the user is not actually involved in the programming, other than to specify which statistical computations are desired from the professional programmer. This increases the efficiency of computer time, but tends to isolate the researcher from an understanding of the computer's capacity and flexibility.

In analyzing the results from computer programs, the student should be cautioned about the adoption of a blind faith in the results, and the more experienced researcher is inclined to use some pencil-and-paper calculations to check a few means, degrees of freedom, F ratios, and other values that may seem a bit too large or too small. The computer's speed, efficiency, and attention to detail are powerful assets to the researcher's efforts, but the computer has no capacity for skepticism or suspicion of errors; these functions must be supplied by the user.

The new user may at first be impressed, or even startled, by the apparently human characteristics of the computer. Programmers, as a group, tend to treat the computer as a somewhat grumpy colleague, who may or may not be in the mood to run a program at any given time. Indeed, the computer does seem to have personality. On some occasions, it may run a program even though it contains a few minor errors. At other times, the program may be aborted because of the same error. In these instances, the programmer may say either that the computer "forgave" our error or "didn't like" the statement. The human image is further enhanced in some computer-assisted study programs, in which the user's correctly typed answer to a question may be greeted with "VERY GOOD, BILL. YOU LEARN QUICKLY. NOW LET'S GO ON TO THE NEXT QUESTION."

Our anthropomorphic treatment of the computer seems to stem not only from its capricious nature, but also from our use of real words to "talk" with the computer. The computer's human characteristics will probably appear even stronger as more models are developed to use spoken messages to replace typewritten material.

OUTLINE OF COMPUTER PROGRAMS

Just as the thesis or dissertation is usually divided into five chapters, with each chapter containing a specific body of information, the computer program normally contains four sections of rather standard information that are organized according to a standardized sequence. In general, the first section identifies the user and the job to be done, the second tells the computer how to do the job, the third gives the computer the data to be used, and the fourth gives the computer the signal to start and finish the job. The style, vocabulary, and punctuation vary from one computer language to the next, but the overall outline is relatively consistent.

Section 1. The Job Control Section

This section contains the information preliminary to getting the system set up to run the job. It includes the user's identification and account number, the job title, estimated running time, and the computer package from which the statistic will be used. From this information, the computer checks the person's identification as a registered user, charges the fee to the proper account, and stores the user's name and job title to be used on the print-out of the results. It retrieves the requested statistical program out of storage to receive the special instructions for treatment of the data, and to receive the data.

Section 2. The Program Instruction Section

At this stage, the statistical variables are identified, the number of columns and rows of data are specified, subtitles are provided for use in the results, and special instructions are given as to what should be included or omitted in the print-out. For example, the user may or may not wish to have the entire program and the raw data listed in the print-out.

If the program is being run for the first time, it is wise to have the entire program and the raw data included in the print-out, because there is usually a need to correct some small error or to modify the program to get further information in a later run.

Section 3. The Data Section

Each set of data is given a title that is used by the computer to retrieve the data set for computation or to rearrange or combine data in any way. Data titles are kept short and often abbreviated, as in H-LOSS, LANG, IQ., or STUTT. The data themselves are always entered in a specific arrangement, such as by rows, so that the computer can find any number by its location. If the data are on punch cards, it is very helpful to have one punch card for each subject, so that subjects may be grouped according to different criteria as needed.

Section 4. The Completion Section

This section is very short, often consisting only of two statements. It signals the computer that all of the program has now been put in and that the computer should start the run and finish at this point. The computer will not begin unless the finish statement is included.

COMMONLY USED COMPUTER SYSTEMS (PACKAGES)

A number of computer systems have been developed for application in various fields of interest, such as business statistics, medical research, and general data processing. Each system, or "package", therefore, has its own language, its own mode of punctuation, and its own strengths and weaknesses as to how well it could meet the user's needs. This complicates problems of gaining familiarity with the computer because the average user in the speech and hearing field will need to draw upon statistics from perhaps three different packages in order to obtain the appropriate treatments for his or her research needs. Unfortunately, we cannot simply choose one system that meets all of our statistical needs, and learn it well enough for general application. Because each system has so many unique aspects, and most systems are revised periodically, the difficulties in becoming a self-sufficient computer user are beyond the time and effort of many researchers.

SPSS "Statistical Programs for the Social Sciences"

This system uses FORTRAN as the computer language, and is frequently revised and updated to incorporate more efficient methods and new statistical treatments that are continually being developed by independent users in the field. It is particularly well-suited to inferential statistics, such as an analysis of variance, but does not have a strong capability in descriptive statistics, such as the presentation of charts, graphs, and similar layouts.

SAS "Statistical Analysis System"

Developed at North Carolina State University, these programs are written in PL/1 language, which means that it is compatible only to IBM computers or those of similar manufacture. It is particularly well-suited for data organization such as layouts, charts, graphs, and other descriptive statistics and summary reports. It is also adequate in most other commonly used statistics, and performs especially well in various kinds of regression analysis.

BMD "Bio Medical Division"

This is the oldest of which might be called the popular statistical packages, developed at the University of California for use in the medical science field. As a general rule, the older the system, the more difficult it is to use, and the original BMD packages were more difficult than the more recent SPSS and SAS systems. It is capable of particularly elaborate types of statistical computations, some of which are considerably beyond the scope of common research needs. It uses FORTRAN language, and is well-suited for very precise types of statistical treatments. An updated version of BMD, known as "BMPD", has a somewhat more streamlined and easier style, but most programmers still consider it to be more difficult to use than some of the other systems.

COMPUTER LANGUAGES

Assembler Language

This is actually a family of computer language that is used by systems programmers, and is not used by application programmers. In other words, assembler language must first be programmed into the machine before it can begin to function as a computer. It is simply a mathematical language that allows the computer to bridge the gap between electronic circuitry and the meaningful functions which can be interpreted by computer users. Each manufacturer of computers uses its own assembler language, which is tailored to the circuitry of their products.

PL/1 "Program Language 1"

This language was developed by IBM for use with IBM-manufactured computers. It is IBM compatable, which means that it can be used only with IBM or similarly designed computers. It is essentially a combination of FORTRAN and COBAL languages. In many respects, it is considered a difficult computer language to learn because it incorporates an extremely expansive variety of symbolization, but this allows an almost unlimited functional capacity and flexibility.

FORTRAN "Formula Translation"

Developed in 1954 as a computer language for scientists and engineers, FORTRAN, with its revised versions, has remained the fundamental scientific research language for most computers. It is not dependent upon any particular manufacture of computer models, and serves very well at all levels of statistical computation. It is, however, not particularly well-suited to graphic presentations, such as charts and layouts associated with descriptive statistics.

COBOL "Common Business Oriented Language"

This language was developed for typical financial and office computer use, such as financial summaries, payroll, personnel, interest rates, and similar business needs. It includes many key words that are used in business statistics and accounting.

BASIC "Beginner's All-purpose Symbolic Instructional Code"

This is the language used by the "home computers" or "minicomputers." It was designed at Dartmouth College to resemble regular English language as closely as possible, and to use common algebraic logic so as to be readily adaptable to the new user. BASIC is well-suited for computerized instruction programs, which are often set up to be available through interuniversity terminals. Although it may contain many of the fundamental statistical computations, such as the t, Pearson r, chi square, and analysis of variance, it is employed mostly in user-generated programs, rather than in the larger commercial statistical packages.

Three modifications of BASIC are currently available. "Pure BASIC" is the original version, developed originally for full sized computers. Microsoft BASIC is a later modification, developed for microcomputers, and will allow for more instructions per line, which is a space-saver for the smaller storage units. Another version, known as TRS BASIC was developed for use by Radio Shack home computers. This is called a *product compatable* language which means that it can be used only in units of a certain manufacture.

A characteristic of this system is that there is very little that is automatic or assumed about its output in comparison to other systems; everything must be specified in the program instructions in order to appear in the results and nothing is taken for granted. On the other hand, the system is relatively robust in terms of user errors, in that some minor user errors will be tolerated, and the system will go on to produce results anyway. This is definitely less frustrating for the beginner, but contains the hazard of printing erroneous results without signaling the presence of mistakes in the program. Finally, where very elaborate computations are to be used with large amounts of data, the BASIC system may be considered as a relatively slow system. For most common statistical problems, however, this difference in computational rate would scarcely be noticed.

Particularly, if BASIC is used in interuniversity program sharing, such as MICC (Middle Illinois Computer Co-op), it is well-suited as an interactive system, which means that it can be used to store and call up other statistical packages according to the changing demands of the user.

PASCAL

A language considered by some to be an expanded version of BASIC is PASCAL, named after the seventeenth century mathematician. This language has the simplicity of BASIC, but the statistical capacity of larger and more complicated systems. As the demand for greater performance in micro- and minicomputers increases, PASCAL may eventually supercede BASIC as the primary language in these smaller sized units.

THE COMPUTERIZED REFERENCE SEARCH

Computer Search Technology

The computer search technique is about the same as looking manually into a shelf reference book, such as *Psychological Abstracts, DSH Abstracts,* or the *Reader's Guide to Periodical Literature.* The main difference is that a computer search can look through a great many references in a few minutes, and print them out complete with abstracts in about a half hour. The same task done manually would usually require several hours or several days in the library, involving tedious reading and the taking of notes. The manual method is still adequate for a term paper or a narrowly specialized research project, but has become "old fashioned" and obsolete as a means of reviewing the literature for a thesis or dissertation. The advantages of the computer search are that it is incredibly fast and thorough, covering more territory of sources than would be available in some libraries, overlooking nothing, and writing out all the citations and abstracts virtually without error. The two disadvantages are that the computer search usually charges a nominal fee (about $10 or $20, although some are free), and that the researcher does not have the luxury of browsing through the literature.

There are two types of requests for the searched material. The quickest method is called the online search or the *interactive* search. This method allows the user to communicate more or less directly with the data base. This gives the user an immediate idea of the amount of material available in his/her first request and allows him/her to judge whether or not to modify the request to include a greater number of years or a greater number of concept terms (called *descriptors*). The references that fit the request are called *hits*. These can be printed out immediately on the user's terminal (online) or are printed out in the system's central computer (offline) and sent air mail to the user. The air mail bibliography is used when there are a relatively larger number of references and abstracts involved in the search. The second type of request is the *batch* method, which is often used for the ERIC search. This method employs hand-written descriptors filled out on a paper form by the user. These forms are accumulated until a group (or "batch") of searches can be made at one time. This search is normally conducted at night when the computer is not busy with other projects, and uses material stored on tape ("mag tapes"), which has been sent by mail to the local computer. Although this method is rather slow, taking one or two weeks to deliver the print-out, it is the cheapest computer search technique, and very satisfactory when delivery time is not crucial

Although some centers encourage direct user participation, most centers are dependent upon a skilled computer librarian to set up the commands for the search and to advise the user. The future trend, however, is to install a *user interface* system, which means that the user may eventually operate a program similar to the computerized teaching method. through a series of steps, the computer will ask the user for topics of interest, need for abstracts, number of citations desired, and types of journals and span of publication years to be included in the search. By this means, an inexperienced researcher could conduct an adequate search without arranging for the services of the computer specialist. With greater volume of use, brought about by this simplification, the relative cost of the searches will probably decline.

Even though the cost of computer searches are nominal, the average student is not in the position to spend an extra $10 or $20 each time a bibliography is needed, and most faculty members are similarly frugal. This, together with the scheduling of program consultation time and facilities, represents the only deterrent to extremely widespread proliferation and routine use of this rapid information gathering technique. At present, some systems, such as the batch search method of the ERIC system, are very cheap or even free to students and faculty. Others, such as MEDLARS and BRS are usually handled at low institutional cost, either at a flat user fee or a low rate based on the number of references obtained through the search. The main systems designed for commercial use, such as Dialog and ORBIT charge a fee based upon the number of references found (hits) plus the amount of computer time consumed in the search. Part of the search fee goes to the index publishing company, which charges a small royalty to the computer system for each title and abstract printed by the computer. Some of the more expensive searches are for the use of data bases in the business, finance, and commercial categories, which also have the capacity to print summary charts and graphs as an additional service.

The main options for the user, as indicated earlier are the topics of interest, the inclusion of abstracts, the maximum number of citations needed, and the types of journals and years to be covered. The topics must usually be chosen from the published list of descriptors used to categorize the data base. These may be used singly or in combination, as in hearing-loss/children. The MEDLARS system is considered to have the most carefully constructed descriptor categories, designed to give a user the maximum opportunity of retrieving all of the desired articles without filling the print-out with un-wanted references. The user's skill in selecting the most accurate descriptors will enhance the efficiency of any of the systems.

Another type of entry used by some search systems is called the "free search." This means that any key word may be supplied by the user, and the computer will scan the titles and abstracts of all references in the data base in order to retrieve everything which contains the key word. A key word might be "lisp", "intelligibility", or "Meniere's", for example.

Nearly all available search systems include the capability to print abstracts as well as references. Part of the abstract capability, however, depends upon whether an abstract appeared with the published article. Most systems allow the user the option of omitting the abstracts, which reduces the cost of retrieval.

In nearly all cases, the user would wish to limit the amount of material to be gathered in the search, because a great deal of unwanted citations only increases the cost and the amount of paper to be handled. For this reason, each system has a number of limiting options, such as "only the most recent 75 items", "only U.S. journals", or "only the last five years." If a comprehensive bibliography is desired for a thesis or dissertation, the full scan may be needed to cover as much scope as possible.

As a final note about reference searches in general, the field of speech, language, and hearing is a particularly difficult and unwieldy area to classify by any existing library reference system. Whereas disciplines like medicine, law, or engineering are relatively well-defined, communicative disorders, to the librarians' dismay, are notoriously spread throughout numerous unrelated areas. Common sources include education, nursing, medicine, psychology, physiology, speech, sociology, and linguistics.

Computer Library Reference Search Systems

The main computer search systems available to most university libraries are ERIC, MEDLARS, ORBIT, Dialog, and BRS. In addition, most university libraries belong to a regional interlibrary information exchange group, which is linked by computer terminals. ERIC deals with educational references, and MEDLARS deals with medical information. ORBIT, Dialog, and BRS are general reference systems that have data bases to cover nearly any major field of interest. The latter three systems are rather similar in use and scope of topics, and preference of any one over the others seems to be mainly a subjective choice. Computer librarians have noticed that many scientists are inclined to use Dialog, while students generally appreciate the cheaper rates of the BRS system.

ERIC

The acronym ERIC stands for Educational Resources Information Center. The information center itself is in Washington, D.C., but there are 13 subcenters, called *information clearinghouses*, which are scattered around the nation. The clearinghouses, mostly located on university campuses, each deal with a certain specialty area, such as "education for the handicapped." Each clearinghouse feeds its current information into the center in Washington, which puts all the combined information on magnetic computer tapes (mag tapes). Current updated tapes are mailed to all participating libraries or other computer reference centers every two weeks. The centers then store the tapes to provide a reference search for anyone needing bibliographic information. In additional to local availability of the magnetic storage tapes, most local institutions can arrange a search of the central ERIC data base. The ERIC system covers most education journals, but sometimes may also include education-related references that the local clearinghouse staff might pick up from other sources. The system is set up to print mainly titles of journal articles, but includes some book titles as well. The search is made by using a two-word combination of descriptors, such as "deafness/children."

These descriptors are listed in the ERIC Thesaurus, which is always available at the local reference center office. Its main compilation sources are *Resources in Education* and *Current Index to Journals in Education.* It can be programmed to print out only a certain time span of references, such as "only the most recent 75 references", etc. This keeps the user's quantity within a more efficient package, and saves time, money, and reduces bulk of unwanted print-out. In addition to the use of descriptors, the ERIC search will also accept the name of a specific author which the user may wish to cite, and will print out all of the references under that author's name.

There are two methods that are available to the user at most ERIC reference centers. The most common is the "batch" retrieval method, which allows the number of requests to accumulate until a small pile or batch is ready. All of the requests are then put at once into the university's computer system, usually during one night of the week when the computer is not too heavily loaded with other types of work. While the batch method is very inexpensive (in some centers, it is free to students and faculty), it has a built-in delay of about a week before a batch of requests accumulates for the next search. A faster but more expensive method is called on *online* search. By this method the national ERIC data base can be reached through another retrieval system, such as *Dialog.*

The ERIC system is not limited to education as it applies to children, but includes all aspects of education, such as adult education, continuing education departments of education, and other categories applied to a wide variety of settings and age levels. Conversely, it does not include medical problems of children or other noneducational aspects of remediation and therapy.

MEDLARS (MEDLINE)

MEDLARS stands for Medical Literature Analysis and Retrieval System. MEDLINE stands for "MEDLARS online." This search system has a data base made from the three main medical index sources: *Index Medicus, International Index of Nursing,* and *Index to Dental Literature.* It is particularly useful for speech and hearing disorders that are medically or hospital oriented, such as laryngectomy, acoustic tumor, or aphasia. It is not applicable for nonmedical areas, such as child language development, speech improvement programs, or hearing screening in the schools.

The indexing system for MEDLARS has been developed by professional medical librarians and is considered to be a very precise and accurate system of subject matter classification. It prints bibliographic reference and the abstracts, particularly if an abstract was included in the original article.

The user may request only the references, without the abstracts. Materials found by the computer may be requested by interlibrary loan from the National Library of Medicine if it is not locally available to the user.

This search system was developed by the National Institutes of Health to service all of the institutes which fall under that bureau. (The speech and hearing area is considered to be within the scope of the National Institute of Neurological and Communicative Disorders and Stroke (NINCDS).) MEDLARS is housed in the National Library of Medicine, in Bethesda, Maryland, and is subscribed only by university libraries which are associated with schools of medicine or schools of nursing. It is key-word oriented and year-oriented, which means that it will search topics or words in articles which were published within a designated span of years.

Dialog (also called Lockheed)

This is a commercially developed computer search system that was originated by a division of the Lockheed Corporation, Lockheed Information Services (LIS), housed in Palo Alto, California. It prints out titles and abstracts, covering reference materials such as Psych Abstracts, DSH Abstracts, and Index Medicus, as well as those in physics, chemistry, and other sciences. Like many other search systems, it can be reached by access terminals that are designed to hold the receiver of any standard desk telephone. The user simply lays the telephone in the computer terminal carriage and types in user identification code which is then cleared for use by the central computer in Palo Alto.

It accepts descriptor terms or author names for any category of information the user intends to search. As with many other search systems, Dialog charges the user by the number of references (hits) supplied to the user, and by the amount of computer time used in the search. A specialized function of this system is in the production of charts or graphs, which are designed to cover certain types of trends or summaries in specialized topics. To date, however, this capacity is used mainly in the business and commercial fields, which are more likely to have such charts in their data base.

BRS

BRS stands for Bibliographic Retrieval Services, which is a commercial computer search system very much like Dialog and ORBIT. It originated within the State University of New York (SUNY) libraries as a general purpose library search system geared to meet the needs of university library reference work and the research interests commonly found in the university setting. As in the other search systems, it prints both citations of articles and abstracts, particularly if the abstracts have been included as part of the original article. BRS is often preferred by graduate students because of its slightly lower user costs. Its data base is frequently revised to include greater scope and depth of material.

SDC (ORBIT)

This system tends to be slightly more complicated to use than are the other systems, but because the user does not actually call up the search program, this is not usually an important consideration. The computer librarian must exercise special care and attention to detail in programming a search from this system. It is from the Systems Development Corporation (SDC), of Santa Monica, California, which also manufactures computers and computer software.

ORBIT is much like the other search systems, such as Dialog and BRS. It has more variety of sources than BRS but is also slightly more expensive. It does not have quite as much selection as Dialog. In addition to the customary descriptor searches ORBIT can run a search which scans for any key word at the first 50 words through the title and summary of any article. It also has the capacity to limit a search to materials from specific cities, states, or countries.

Also associated with SDC is a system called SSIE, Smithsonian Science Information Exchange. This is primarily an on-line search of funded research projects which are currently in progress or which have been completed during the past two years. The data base covers about 200,000 projects, with 60% in the life science fields and 40% in the physical sciences. The print-out identifies the projects and gives a 200 word summary of each. Descriptors for this system are arranged in order from broad concepts to narrow concepts, which allows for a rather large group of citations listed under broad headings or a very specific few listings which would appear under narrowly defined headings.

Regional Library Search Networks

It is common for groups of libraries in any given state or other geographical region to participate in an interlibrary exchange system, somewhat like the familiar interlibrary loan system. These are particularly useful for university libraries. Fundamentally, these systems represent a sharing of each other's card files, or other reference information. In most cases, these systems are used routinely by the library staff, rather than by the specific individual user who may be looking for a certain book or reference. In fact, in routine situations, the individual user is unaware that the interlibrary search system is being used to find the particular citation. These systems are usually designated by names which end in the letters "NET", such as MIDLNET, which is the midwest network, or "NELINET" for the New England states network.

Although the system is typically set up as an interlibrary exchange, most of these systems also subscribe to the main large periodical search data bases as well, such as BRS, ORBIT, and Dialog.

PART 2

Statistical Treatment

CHAPTER 7　Preliminary Planning for Statistical Treatment

One who attempts to advise students as to the most appropriate statistical treatments is apt to be confronted with questions such as, "What is the simplest statistic I can possibly use?"; "Could I just use t-tests for everything, instead of an analysis of variance?"; or "Now that I have collected my data, what statistic should I use?" These questions, although exasperating, convey the unfortunate predicament of the student attempting to learn scientific methodology. In spite of the long history of statistical requirements in the speech and hearing curriculum, the traditional approach to this subject has failed notoriously to serve its purpose. Although some blame may go the insensitive instruction of dry statistical material, other contributing factors probably include too long a time lapse between course and application, and a general tendency to view research as being entirely separate from clinical interests.

Statistics books as a group are plagued by a lack of uniformity in notation from one author to the next. For the student with only a moderate mathematical background, the array of statistical symbols could rival the hieroglyphics of Egyptian tombs. Even for the experienced researcher, the most worn pages in statistical references are the worked examples of various types of problems. The need for simplification in statistical references is further illustrated by the remarkable success of what is informally called a "statistical cookbook" by Bruning and Kintz (1977). This is not to debate the merits of sound mathematical insight into statistical computation, but rather to acknowledge certain deficiencies in our traditional approach to research training.

Three basic texts appear most often on the reference shelf, as indicated by the bibliographies from journal articles in the speech, language, and hearing area:

Winer, B., *Statistical Principles of Experimental Design*. New York: McGraw-Hill, 1971.

Siegel, S., *Nonparametric Statistics for the Behavioral Sciences*. New York: McGraw-Hill, 1956.

Bruning, J., and Kintz, B., *Computational Handbook of Statistics*. Glenview, Ill.: Scott Foresman, 1977.

For the majority of statistical problems, the combination of these three texts will be found well worth the investment, both in terms of computational guidance and in explanation of the assumptions which underlie each treatment. Other commonly used statistical references include:

Lindquist, E., *Design and Analysis of Experiments in Psychology and Education*. New York: Houghton Mifflin, 1953.

Myers, J., *Fundamentals of Experimental Design*. New York: Allyn and Bacon, 1972.

Guilford, J., *Fundamental Statistics in Psychology and Education*. New York: McGraw-Hill, 1956.

Ferguson, G., *Statistical Analysis in Psychology and Education*. New York: McGraw-Hill, 1971.

Steele, R., and Torrie, J., *Principles and Procedures of Statistics*. New York: McGraw-Hill, 1960.

Kirk, R., *Experimental Design: Procedures for the Behavioral Sciences*. Belmont, Cal.: Brooks-Cole, 1968.

ANSWERING QUESTIONS WITH STATISTICS

A common pitfall of the uninitiated researcher is in formulating questions which literally cannot be answered through investigative techniques. The language of research findings is in the form of numbers. Sometimes the numbers are very simple, as in the average number of stutterers in clinicians' caseloads, and at other times the numbers are very complex, as in the computer print-out for a three factor analysis, but they are always in the form of numbers. To decide whether or not the research question is actually answerable, therefore, the student must ask himself or herself what sort of numbers will provide the answer. One helpful technique is to pose all research questions to conclude with the phrase "as determined by. . . . " This type of phrasing gives the question a built-in criterion for determining the answer, as in the question "Is there a difference in speaker anxiety between stutterers and nonstutterers, as determined by skin response amplitude?" In this case, the measure of skin response amplitude will be the criterion for whether or not a difference exists between the two groups. From this point, it is a simple matter to project the type of data which will be used and the specific statistical treatment which should be applied.

Another practical way to think about research questions is to phrase each question so that it may be answered either with "yes" or "no." This wording implies that the answer will be specified as "yes, the difference is significant", or "no, the difference was not significant." For example, "Is there a difference in language test scores between preschool boys and girls?"

A poor research question, statistically speaking, would be, "How does language develop among inner city children?" Although the topic would appear to be timely, important, and interesting, it does not contain criteria for defining the variables or for knowing whether or not the question has been answered. This type of question is very helpful in the initial stages of planning the research project or for general discussion at the end of the report, but does not lend itself to a statistical answer.

Although we need not actually write out a series of research questions in order to arrive at the final draft, it will be helpful to follow the development of some typical research concepts, from the initial general idea to the final hypothesis. In nearly all of the cases, the thought process evolves through three stages. The initial stage merely defines the area of interest, the second stage defines the variables to be observed, and the third stage defines the hypothesis to be tested.

Stage I: Defining the General Area of Interest:

The initial phase of planning is to form some broad concept of the topical area or of the general purpose of the study. The question itself may be only implied, and is usually made in informal conversational terms. Ideally, the student should come to the thesis or dissertation advisor with at least an informal hypothesis, but in practice this is rarely the case. It is not unusual for the initial idea to be expressed as, "I would like to do a thesis on Black language," or "What would you think about a study on evoked response and loudness?", or even more generally, "I am planning to do something either in stuttering or voice." All of these statements contain at least the germ of a future hypothesis, but are still too vague for research application. The more experienced doctoral student may be able to conceive the entire project by himself/herself, but most others need guidance from those more familiar with current issues and trends in the areas of interest. Although it is poor practice for the advisor to assume so much of the planning that the student becomes somewhat of a bystander, it is important for the student to be thoughtfully advised and steered in the proper direction by those with special insight into the proposed topic. This is especially beneficial to the early formative stage of planning.

Stage II: Defining the Variables to be Observed:

After the topic has been described informally, the variables and the specific type of data should be visualized. This is perhaps the most difficult level of questions to formulate because it represents the main transition from the informal concept to a more structured research design. Implicit in the definition of variables is their classification as to the dependent and independent role in the study. One aspect of the difficulty is that the same concept may be treated effectively by several different techniques. In the example mentioned previously, the study on loudness and evoked response might be set up as a comparison between two groups of data—the loud stimulus group vs. the soft stimulus group. It might just as easily be treated as a correlation between relative sound intensity and evoked response amplitude. In many instances the choice of design is more or less arbitrary, since the point of the study can be shown by several different methods. One soon finds that no two advisors recommend exactly the same experimental design. At this stage the student is vulnerable to conflicting advice, and a dilemma may develop over trying to find the "best" way to set up the study. In many instances there is no "best" way; it is simply a matter of how the investigator feels the results should be presented. This type of problem should be resolved in the prospectus meeting or should be worked out individually with the thesis advisor.

The variables and the data should be kept as simple as possible, and should not be left vague and complicated. In audiology, for example, the most familiar variables are intensity, frequency, and standardized verbal material. The numerical data are typically in the form of thresholds or discrimination scores. In stuttering, the variables might include the type of speech material or situation, and the data are the number of blocks counted by judges, while language and articulation studies can rely upon standardized verbal test scores.

Stage III: Stating the Working Hypothesis and the Null Hypothesis:

The final level of refinement for the research concept is putting each question into a form which can be answered specifically in terms of statistical results. As a general rule, these questions (or statements) are stated clearly at the end of the Introduction section of the research report, and are used later to form the outline for the statistical presentation in the Results section. The working hypothesis is actually in the form of a question, whereas the null hypothesis is worded in the form of a negative statement which conveys an implied question.

The working hypothesis asks the research question in the researcher's own language; it expresses the project in the way the researcher is actually thinking about it, as in "Will evoked response amplitude increase as stimulus loudness increases?" or "Is Black language development affected by socio-economic level?" Each of these questions expresses the independent and dependent variable, and each can be answered with a "yes" or "no" according to the significance or nonsignificance of a statistical result. It should also be noted that each of these topics will produce acceptable contributions regardless of whether the results are significant or not.

The null hypothesis may or may not actually be stated in a published article, but it is almost always required for the thesis and dissertation. It is written in the language of statistical logic, which states that nothing has really happened unless proven otherwise. Nearly all null hypotheses begin with the words "There is no difference between . . . ", or "There is no relationship between. . . . " Through this wording, the burden of proof is placed upon the investigator, and if the investigator cannot show a significant difference or relationship, these events are dismissed as probable coincidence. From the previous examples, the formal null hypotheses would read, "There is no relationship between evoked response amplitude and sound stimulus intensity" or "There is no difference between language test results from two socio-economic groups of 4-year-old Black children."

Particularly in the thesis or dissertation, the statistical result is stated in terms of whether or not the null hypothesis can be rejected. In published reports and articles, as mentioned earlier, although the null hypothesis is always implied, it is not necessarily stated in full.

To a great extent the wording of the research question suggests not only the type of data but also the treatment which will be used. Here are some additional examples:

"Is there a significant correlation between a standardized language screening test and the new screening test for preschool children?" This question points toward the use of a correlation technique, such as the Pearson "r" or the Spearman "rho."

"What is the percentage of agreement between the two articulation screening tests, as applied to preschool children?" A question which refers to percentages may not suggest a computational formula but rather that the percentage itself may be the result. Since there is no level of significance in this type of result, it is called a *descriptive statistic.*

"Is there a significant difference between language screening test scores and standard test scores among the three age groups?" The answer to this kind of question would be derived most likely through an analysis of variance, because more than two groups of data are presented.

Through the foregoing discussion, it may be seen that once the preliminary thinking has narrowed the investigation into a series of well-defined questions, the exact nature of the data arrangement becomes clear, leaving little chance for later confusion. Given a well-defined hypothesis, the choice of statistical treatment becomes a simple matter.

CHOOSING THE APPROPRIATE STATISTIC

For the thesis advisor, a student who has completed the statistics requirements but cannot apply the techniques to a real research problem represents an old story and one which is often repeated. The problem lies not in the lack of academic achievement but rather in a lack of experience with applied methods. The following presentation outlines the principles of statistical application as a series of choices which the more experienced researcher may utilize intuitively. Those who are still developing their applied skills, however, should find the choices and the rationale for each choice to be an insightful simplification of some forgotten statistical concepts.

Within the framework of the most commonly applied statistical treatments, the chart which appears at the beginning of the statistical worked examples serves to categorize the formulas appropriate for the basic types of experimental designs. The chart is based upon an understanding of four fundamental classifications for evaluating groups of data:

1. Number of groups: Are there two groups, or more than two groups?
2. Relationship of the groups: Are the groups composed of independent or related measures?
3. Distribution of data: Is the distribution normal, nonparametric, or binomial?
4. Type of result stated in the hypothesis: Are the results to be in terms of comparison or relationship between groups?

1. Number of Groups in the Study

The key question under this heading is "Are there two groups or more than two groups to be considered in the study?" The whole gamut of statistical treatments can be divided arbitrarily into those which are designed for use with only two groups and those which are for more than two groups. Most familiarly, the two group category of statistics would include the t-test and the multiple group category might involve an analysis of variance. As a generalization, two-group statistics are usually easier and less complicated to compute than are multiple group statistics, partly because of the sheer difference in the number of groups, but also because two-group statistics also include some very common nonparametric techniques. Since nonparametrics employ rank order transformations and tally counts, the arithmetic involves smaller numbers and much less computation. Although many multiple group statistics can be computed on the hand calculator, the use of squared values and cross-multiplications make the more elaborate versions impossible from a practical standpoint by any means except the computer.

As a very simple illustration in the number of data groups, if we were to give articulation tests to our case load of children before and after a period of speech therapy, this would represent a two-group study. If we were to test the children before, at midterm, and after therapy, this would involve three groups, or, in other words, a multiple group study.

Comparisons Between Two Groups of Data

Most research projects are based primarily upon the comparison of two groups of data. Clinical studies, for instance, are often based upon some difference between a clinical group as compared with an equivalent group of normals. A typical study of this nature is reported by Dworkin (1978), who compared lingual force of lispers and normal speakers. A t-test between the two groups indicated that lispers have significantly less force and mobility of the tongue than was found in normal speakers.

The t-test is generally considered to be the heart of the simple two-group comparison design, and other tests are sometimes explained in terms of the t-test analogy. As a general rule, then, when we consider comparing two groups, we are likely to think first of the t-test, because it is a very common choice. However, several questions need to be asked first before the final choice is made. The first is to ask whether the comparison is to be made between two separate groups of subjects—as in lispers and normals—or are the same subjects used for both measures, as in testing a group before and after therapy? There are two fundamental versions of the t-test. The first is to be used for independent groups, such as lispers and normal speakers, and the second version of the t-test is to used if the same subjects are measured twice. This latter version is called the t-test for related (or correlated) measures. The main distinction is that if all the data are from the same group of subjects, a smaller difference is more likely to be significant.

Using these two versions of the t-test as our basic model, we need to ask next whether our data are normally distributed. There are special tests to check for normal distribution, e.g., Bartlet's Test, but this is usually not a matter of critical importance. As discussed by Winer (1971), moderate departures from normally distributed data do not seriously hamper the accuracy of the t-test. Secondly, the chances are that a sample of scores taken from a representative population will approximate the true distribution. It is only when there is reason to believe that the data are not normally distributed that an alternative to the t-test should be used. Finally, (Hays, 1973) tests used for determining normal distribution tend to break down under small samples and are therefore not worth the additional computation. In other words, tests for determining normalcy are not particularly helpful. The alternate should be chosen: (1) if the scores are closely packed, with no indication of range or variance; (2) if there are so few scores that there is no semblance of a mean or central tendency; (3) or if the data are not in the form of measures or scores, but rather in the form rank order, pass-fail judgments, or similar classifications.

As suggested in the previous discussion, the t-test is the preferred first choice for the comparison of two groups because it is a relatively simple statistic to compute, because it is based upon the validity and confidence intervals of normally distributed samples, and because it is considered to be *robust*—that is, not easily affected by sample size or minor variations in distribution. However, if the t-test should be considered inappropriate because of the nature of the data, two "nonparametric" tests are used as effective analogies of the two basic kinds of t-tests. With independent measures, the nonparametric statistic to use for comparisons is the Mann-Whitney U test. In a study of acoustic reflex thresholds for stutterers and nonstutterers, the narrow spread of the data values in combination with the small N (nine subjects in each group) did not appear as normal distributions, and since all thresholds were similar, the rank order of scores became more important than the means. The Mann-Whitney U results indicated that no differences appeared between the reflex thresholds of the two independent groups of subjects (Horovitz *et al.*, 1978). In the same study, the alternative to the t-test for related measures—the Wilcoxon T—was used to test for difference in acoustic reflex for one group under two conditions (with and without anxiety). The T result indicated significantly lower reflex thresholds for stutterers under the condition of anxiety. The Wilcoxon T was used because both sets of measures were taken from the same group of subjects.

Two additional tests which can be used to check for differences between two groups are the Sign Test and the Difference Between Proportions Test. These two nonparametric techniques are not as widely used as those mentioned previously, but are recommended for special circumstances. The Sign Test is helpful in studies involving listener judgments of paired items, in which one decision is made for each pair. This type of experiment is sometimes found in experimental phonetics, in which each listener is to judge which of two speech sounds seems to be rougher, more nasal, louder, higher, longer, etc. It is therefore considered to be an appropriate test for binomial (plus-minus) data.

The last test to be mentioned in the category of differences between two groups is the Proportions Test. This test is included because of its convenience in testing to see whether a trait appears in proportionately more males than females, or that a response appears proportionately more often in one situation than in another. It is based upon the presence or absence of a certain trait or characteristic among two groups of items.

To summarize the statistics for use with two groups (correlations are described in a later section):
Comparison Between Two Groups:
Independent Groups
Normal Distribution: t-test
Ranked Data: Mann-Whitney U
Related Measures
Normal Distribution: t-test for related measures
Ranked Data: Wilcoxon Matched Pairs T
Binomial Data: Proportions Test
                  Binomial Test

Comparisons with more than Two Groups

The immediate inference to be drawn from the fact that the study is to include more than two groups of data is that some version of the analysis of variance will probably be used. There are three reasons for selecting the analysis of variance, as opposed to the use of separate two-group statistics:

1. The analysis of variance puts all the variables together into one large statistic, rather than a series of smaller computational procedures, and is therefore more efficient, and provides a more compact and easily visualized overall experimental design.

2. The probability is at least theoretically better by using one statistic rather than separate smaller ones. Using a series of t-tests, for example,

increases the probability of statistical error with each additional test used. With one analysis of variance, the chance for error remains the same, regardless of the number of groups in the computation.

3. When several factors are incorporated into the overall design, the analysis of variance adds an additional dimension—interactions—which might not otherwise be included in the treatment. Interactions refer to the manner in which groups of subjects sometimes perform differently (i.e., inconsistently) from each other on different tests. Deaf children, for instance, might score lower than normals on a vocabulary test, but score higher than normals in manual dexterity. This would cause a significant interaction to appear in the groups-by-treatments part of the analysis of variance.

In addition to the analysis of variance, sometimes designated simply as the F test, two other types of tests are available which are suited for multiple-group comparisons. The first are the nonparametric versions of the analysis of variance, which include the Friedman Test, the Kruskal-Wallis H, and the Cochran Q test. In some texts these are also classified as analyses of variance, but in practice are treated as a somewhat separate class of computation.

Comparisons Among Multiple Groups:

Independent Groups

Normal Distribution: One-way analysis of variance (F Test) or factorial analysis of variance for independent measures.

Ranked Data: Kruskal-Wallis H

Repeated Measures

Normal Distribution: Treatments-by-subjects analysis of variance, or factorial analysis of variance with repeated measures on one or more factors.

Ranked Data: Friedman's Test

Binomial Data: Cochran's Q

2. Relationship of the Data Groups: Are the Measures Independent or Related?

A further aspect of comparative statistics depends upon whether or not the groups of scores are derived from separate independent sources. In most cases the criterion for independent measures is that each measure was made from a different group of people. If the same group of people takes two or more tests, the scores are called *dependent measures, related measures,* or sometimes *correlated measures.* For computational purposes all three terms mean the same thing, but the term *correlated measures* points out the underlying statistical characteristic between independent and related measures. If a general relationship or correlation can be assumed among the groups of data, the variances for the two groups will be more homogeneous, making the comparison formula more efficient. Also, the degrees of freedom for related measures tests will be smaller, being based upon the number of *pairs* of scores rather than the combined total. Strictly speaking, related measures need not come from the same population, provided a relationship (i.e., correlation) can be shown. In nearly all cases, however, related measures are derived from the same subjects.

The t-test has two versions, one for independent measures and one for related measures. The nonparametric counterparts for the two t-tests are the Mann-Whitney U and Wilcoxon T test. In the same fashion the one-way analysis of variance is for independent measures and the treatments-by-subjects analysis uses repeated measures. Friedman's Test and the Kruskal-Wallis H are their nonparametric counterparts.

3. Distribution of the Data: Are the Distributions Normal, Nonparametric, or Binomial?

The classifications of the various distributions are discussed in detail in other parts of this text, so that the full descriptions need not be included here. The main consideration, however, is that the three kinds of data relate to three separate classes of statistics.

Data which have a normal distribution must be used with statistics which assume that the scores have a valid standard deviation, or in other words, that if the mean is computed it may be assumed that the majority of the other scores are also in that same general area. If the majority of scores are found not to cluster about the mean, a different group of statistics have been devised which allow for any kind of spread in the group distribution. All that one needs to assume about nonparametric groups of data is that each score will have a different value than the next, since most nonparametric tests use ranked data. The only type of scores which will not fit into this general distribution are tied scores. As a rule, tied scores do not contribute to rank order data, and are often discarded from the computation.

Little has been said up to this point about *binomial data*, which also require a certain method of statistical treatments. This type of data is actually a subdivision of a larger category, called *nominal data*, which refers to the technique of scoring or tallying each result according to a *name* instead of a number. In hearing screening, for example, instead of recording a threshold result of 15 dB, we would simply record the term "pass." All of the resulting tests in the survey would then be recorded either "pass" or "fail." This is an example of binomial data, which means that all scores are placed into one of two classifications. Binomial tests of the difference between two groups of data are the Proportions Test, the Sign Test, and the Binomial Test. With more than two groups, the Chi Square and the Cochran's Q are appropriate.

Since there are only two classifications, binomial data is also called *dichotomous data* in some texts. As implied in the example mentioned previously, other types of measures are sometimes transformed into binomial data, simply by converting all scores into two classes. For instance, children scoring in the upper half of a language test may be called "High;" those in the lower half could be called "Low."

4. Type of Conclusion Stated in the Hypothesis: Does the study intend to *Compare* Groups or to Determine *Relationships* Between Groups?

Most statistical formulas are for the purpose of comparisons; that is, to determine whether one group of scores is significantly larger than another group. In other instances, however, the purpose of the study is to test for a *relationship* or correlation between groups of data. It is not unusual for some studies to require both comparisons and relationships in deriving the conclusions. As discussed earlier, statistics used for the comparison of two or more groups include the t, analysis of variance, Friedman's test, the Kruskal-Wallis H, the Mann-Whitney U, and the Wilcoxon T.

Statistics about relationships are more commonly referred to as correlations.

Correlations are frequently used, but not particularly well understood. As a rule, the approach is to deal with correlations which are either very low, which we consider to be "insignificant," or with correlations which are very high, which we consider to be "significant." Actually this assumption is statistically false; both high and low correlations may be significant. In fact, if there are 1000 pairs of scores, *any* correlation at all will be found significant. The concept of significance in correlations, therefore, is not particularly helpful. A helpful characteristic, however, of the correlation coefficient is that if it is squared (R^2), it becomes an indicator of the percentage of scores which can be predicted from one group to the other. From this we can see that any correlation less than .70 ($R^2 = 49\%$) will account for less than 50 % of the data. The R^2 concept is being used with increasing frequency and is generally more helpful in interpretation of correlations than is the concept of statistical significance.

Strictly speaking, a correlation implies that each score in one group should have a counterpart which appears in about the same place in a second group of scores. In the case of the two-way chi square, however, no such individual alignment appears because all scores are binomial. This statistic, therefore, is more often termed a *relationship* rather than an actual correlation.

One of the clearest examples of research based upon the correlation between two sets of data is a study by Hollien (1960), in which it was demonstrated that as the vocal pitch becomes higher, the vocal chords become thinner. When two kinds of measures are found to be related, it then becomes possible to predict one measure from the other. For instance, when a child's age is known it becomes possible to estimate his approximate language test score. Correlated measures may be either positively or negatively related. That is, both related scores may get larger together, or one may get larger as the other gets smaller. In this sense, a child's age and vocabulary would be positively correlated, while age and articulation errors would be negatively correlated. The most familiar correlational statistic is the Correlation Coefficient, otherwise known as the Pearson Product Moment, or simply the Pearson r.

In summary, the most common statistics to show relationships (correlations) between groups of data are:

Correlations for Two Groups
    Normal Distribution: Pearson r
    Ranked Data: Spearman Rho
    Binomial Data: Two-by-two Chi Square
Correlations Among Several Groups
    (These normally require computer programs, and are not included in this text.)
    Multiple Correlation
    Multiple Regression

The Decision-Making Process for Statistical Treatment

In the following article:

Murry, T., Speaker fundamental frequency characteristics associated with voice pathologies. *J. Speech Hearing Dis.*, 43, 374–379, 1978,

the abstract begins:

"This study investigated the relationship between pathologic and normal speaking fundamental frequency characteristics (SFF) in a group of 80 male subjects. The subjects were divided into four groups of 20 (1) vocal paralysis, (2) benign mass lesion, (3) cancer of the larynx, and (4) normal."

(Murry, 1978, p. 374)

Table 7.1 Criteria for statistical treatments

Type of Data	Comparisons between Groups		Correlations
	Independent Groups	Related Measures	
Analysis for Two Groups			
Normal Distribution	t-Test for Independent Groups	t-Test for Related Measures	Pearson r Correlation Coefficient
Nonparametric Ranks	Mann-Whitney U	Wilcoxon Matched Pairs T	Spearman RHO
Binomial	Proportions Test* z	Sign Test z Binomial Test	Two-Way Chi Square X^2
Analysis for Several Measures of One Factor			
Normal Distribution	One Way Analysis of Variance F	Treatments-by-Subjects Analysis of Variance F	
Nonparametric Ranks	Kruskal-Wallis H	Friedman Test X^2	
Binc.	Chi Square X^2	Cochran Q	
Analysis for Multiple Factors	Randomized Blocks Analysis of Variance F	Factor Analysis with Repeated Measures F	

* Can be independent or related measures.

If we were to decide which statistic would be appropriately used, our comprehensive series of questions can be asked in order to arrive at a reasonable solution. It should be mentioned also at this point that a rearrangement of data, or a change in the slant of the hypothesis could change the criteria for the statistics to be used.

1. Are there two groups or more than two groups? There are four voice types in the study, with each group containing 20 subjects. Therefore, the results are to be based upon *more than two groups* (4) of data.

2. Are the groups independent or related? Each set of scores (Speaking Fundamental Frequency) were obtained from a different group of subjects, rather than using one group of subjects under four test conditions. The data are therefore composed of *independent measures.*

3. Is the distribution normal, nonparametric (ranked), or binomial? This is sometimes a subjective feature, since continuous data can easily be transformed into ranked or binomial data. In this case the fundamental frequency scores for each group were obtained from 20 subjects, which would ordinarily yield a

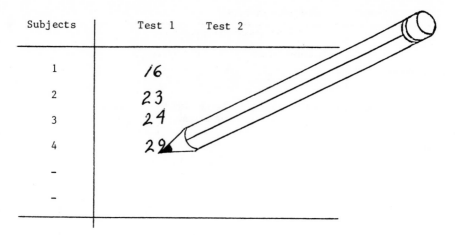

Subjects	Test 1	Test 2
1	16	
2	23	
3	24	
4	29	
–		
–		

Figure 7.1. Data sheet for two groups of data (one factor).

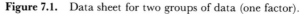

Subjects	Test 1	Test 2	Test 3
Group A			
1			
2			
3			
4			
5			
Group B			
1			
2			
3			
4			
5			

Figure 7.2. Data sheet for a multiple group design (two factors).

representative mean and standard deviation. These data would be considered *normally distributed*.

4. Is the result to compare groups or to show a correlation between groups of scores? The title of the article implies that the purpose was to test for differences among the four vocal types. Therefore, the statistic is to show *comparisons*.

To summarize, Murry (1978) needed a statistical treatment which would

Subjects	Condition I		Condition II	
	Test 1	Test 2	Test 1	Test 2
Group A				
1				
2				
3				
4				
5				
Group B				
1				
2				
3				
4				
5				

Figure 7.3. Data sheet for a multiple factor design (three factors).

encompass more than two groups of data, normally distributed, using independent measures, to test for comparisons. In viewing our chart, which follows, we find that the only statistic which fits the criteria derived from the four questions is the *one-way analysis of variance F test*. On the basis of the F test result, Murry reported a significant difference in vocal fluctuation among the four groups, with the greatest difference appearing between normals and the vocal paralysis group.

THE EXPERIMENTAL DESIGN

As discussed earlier, an essential part of good research planning is to lay out the general pattern of treatment for the data before the project is started. Too often the aspect of data arrangement is overlooked in the planning stage, on the assumption that the data will fall naturally into place at the proper time. Even with relatively simple designs, a collection of unorganized raw data tabulated on various pieces of paper tends to add confusion and even extra work to the proposed statistical treatment. The most expeditious way to set up the data pattern is in the form of a chart from which the computation can be made with clarity and efficiency. Once the data chart is set up, the appropriate arrangement of test scores or other measures is clearly pictured.

When the data are obtained, they can simply be added to the appropriate rows and columns with little chance for confusion or misarrangement.

The charts which follow typify patterns of score sheets for several levels of experimental designs. The first chart (Fig. 7.1) would apply to a wide variety of two-group studies. A common example would be a test-retest design in which a group of subjects might be tested with and without hearing aids, or a group of children might be tested to compare two different articulation screening methods.

The second chart (Fig. 7.2) illustrates a somewhat more complicated design, in which subjects with different types of hearing loss might be tested under several kinds of background noise, or where stutterers and nonstutterers would be evaluated under different speaking conditions.

The last chart (Fig. 7.3) shows how additional variables may be added to the basic design, in instances where multiple factors must be compared in one analysis. Although this particular chart illustrates a three-factor design, additional factors may be stacked up in the same general arrangement. Multiple factor designs of this nature may appear in language studies, in which several age groups at different schools might be administered a number of language subtests.

CHAPTER 8   Descriptive Statistics

Within the total consideration of statistical results it should be kept in mind that not all results involve elaborate statistical computation or even statistical significance. Many types of data are simply a report of the incidence of a certain disorder or characteristic, or else a result which is unique to each individual and should therefore not be reported as an average measure for the population. Most surveys, for example, are designed to report the incidence of some phenomenon, such as the incidence of hearing loss in musicians, and the results are reported simply as percentages. Particularly in speech science, a study may be designed to show individual differences rather than population averages, and this type of result is described on a subject-by-subject basis. When the reader is asked to draw conclusions from percentages, tally counts, or charts showing raw data, means, and standard deviations, the results are called *descriptive statistics*. A review of research journals in the speech and hearing field reveals a remarkably large proportion of studies presented in this manner.

PERCENTAGES

Particularly in clinical studies or surveys, the percentages of subjects' responses becomes the result in itself. Statistically significant differences or correlations between measures are not always the point of the investigation, especially where conclusions can be drawn from a simple summary of the data. The following is a descriptive result from a clinical investigation of middle ear pressure in children:

Although the literature indicated an expected pressure change of approximately 20 mm, only 22 % of the ears tested in the present study demonstrated a middle ear pressure change = 20 mm. Thirty-four percent of the ears evaluated demonstrated no change in middle ear pressure following test procedures.

(Seidemann and Givens, 1977, p. 490)

Although percentages may be used descriptively to report nearly any type of information, the widest use of percentage results is found in surveys. With relatively few percentages to be reported, summary tables and charts are not needed.

Of the children referred over a two-year period, 57 % were found to have vocal nodules; of these, 60 % were bilateral. . . . Slightly more boys (55 %) than girls were referred to the voice clinics. Thirty-six percent of all cases had normal vocal cords, and in 7 % this factor could not be determined because of a strong gag reflex or similar difficulties.

(Shearer, 1972, p. 220)

THE USE OF MEANS AND STANDARD DEVIATIONS

Unlike the use of percentages in descriptive results, means and standard deviations are not commonly used to stand alone. Although these measures could be used by themselves, they are usually preliminary to the use of more computational statistics, such as t-tests or analysis of variance. This type of table may be found in studies in which the results could be used as normative data for comparison with future investigations. In this study the temporary threshold shifts from noise exposure in simulated work conditions were tested. Yates *et al.* (1976) concluded that the 85 dBA noise exposure effects for a full day is significantly less than an equivalent exposure to 90 dBA noise, as part of the analysis of variance results.

Use of Means and Reference to Graphic Display

For the deaf subjects, the average frequency change during the first 120 msec. of the vowel is 160 Hz in one syllable /di/ and 320 Hz in the syllable /bi/. These values are less than half the values for the normal-hearing subjects— 380 and 705 Hz, respectively.

(Monsen, 1976, p. 287)

Monsen (1976) referred to curves made from averaged spectogram values to show the difference between second formant changes in deaf and normal speakers. Results pointed out the difference between the two groups of speakers in terms of the spectographic summaries. Deaf speakers were found to have substantially less frequency change in their transitions between consonants and vowels.

Standard Deviation

In addition to being a part of some statistical formulas, the standard deviation is sometimes reported as a separate statistic in order to explain the variation in scores. The smaller the standard deviation, the closer the scores are to each other, and the more homogeneous is the sample.

Means and standard deviations for the measures of vowel samples as to both horizontal and vertical movement of the hyoid bone are shown in Table 1 and Table 2. It should be noted that more than half of the sample means have a standard deviation of zero, indicating that in most cases all five measures in the sample were indentical.

(Menon and Shearer, 1971, p. 859)

DESCRIPTIONS OF INDIVIDUAL SUBJECT'S RESULTS

Particularly where there are a very small number of subjects used in the study, and the data from each subject are relatively unique, to the extent that the subjects cannot be described realistically as a group, the results from each subject must be described separately. Prosek *et al.* (1978) described the results of biofeedback therapy for six subjects who had functional voice disorders: (p. 286)

Figure 3 presents the data obtained from a 22-year-old female with contact ulcers of the vocal folds. . . . The figure reveals a very orderly reduction in mean EMG activity across sessions with discontinuities occurring, for the most part, only when the speech material was changed.

After each subject is described individually, some generalization should be made by way of conclusions:

The data in Figures 3–8 demonstrate that EMG biofeedback can be used successfully with some patients to alter the level of muscular activity used to produce speech with a concomitant improvement in voice quality.

(*ibid.*, p. 292)

USE OF CHARTS AND GRAPHS TO SUMMARIZE RAW DATA

In the following example, the reader is asked to review a table of raw data which marks the presence or absence of various semantic relations found in the spontaneous language samples from three age groups of children. In this example four aspects of the study result in data which do not conform well to statistical treatment:

1. The data were in the form of binomial (presence vs. absence of the trait) scores, which do not readily represent normal distribution.

2. The N is very small—four children per group.

3. The number of categories—11 semantic relations categories is rather large.

4. A number of the categories contained zero responses, which are not suited to numerical computation. The data were therefore presented in the form of summary tables from which the reader may draw certain conclusions. Considering all aspects, any attempt at statistical treatment would have been awkward at best, and the preferred method was therefore to share the data with the reader instead of forcing a statistical result:

As seen in the table, all 11 semantic relations described by Brown were present in at least one of the sbujects. However, while all relations were observed in the sample, their presence differed across subjects.

(Mallory and Chapman, 1978, p. 207)

At other times the presentation of raw data summaries is used by the investigator to show that it is premature to make strong generalizations at this point, but that some trends show a promising direction for future research.

The composition of charts and graphs to illustrate descriptive results is literally unlimited. Characteristically, audiological studies depict audiograms, articulation and language developmental studies display trend charts or histograms, and studies in acoustic phonetics show scatter diagrams of clustered phonemes. Only a few relatively standard figures are shown here. All tables, charts, and graphs should include a caption which designates the information being presented.

Histograms

The most common use of the histogram is to compare the scores of two or more populations under several related conditions. Although this technique may be used to show trends, its visual impression is to emphasize the values for each fixed measuring condition. The vertical scale (ordinate) of the histogram is usually to represent some measure of achievement such as percentage of correct responses or developmental test scores. The horizontal dimension (abscissa) is used to show different categories which are being measured, such as language subtests, ages, or hearing frequencies. In setting up histograms and similar graphs and charts it is recommended that the ordinate should be about three-fourths the length of the abscissa, in order that a relatively standard sense of perspective is maintained.

The following histogram is similar to a graph presented in a study by Austin (1975), in which the comprehension of various concepts was evaluated by different age groups of a young adult deaf population. On the basis of the concept *vocational comprehension* results the author concluded that educational programs for the deaf should be augmented by greater emphasis in real life experiences. In the following histogram (Fig. 8.1), using simulated data, it is readily seen that conceptual development for the hearing impaired groups lags behind that of the normal hearing population, as described in the study.

Frequency Polygons

The frequency polygon is set up the same as the histogram, but is used to emphasize the aspect of trends in the data. It is composed of dots or similar small geometric marks which are linked by connecting lines. If several populations are shown in the same graph, each is designated by its own geometric figure. When each dot represents a mean value, the standard deviation is sometimes added in the form of a vertical bar which runs through each mean. By far the most common form of the frequency polygon in the speech, language, and hearing field is the audiogram. Other common examples may be found in the adaptation curves for stuttering blocks, and in graphs showing improvement trends throughout certain periods of therapy or rehabilitation programs.

The frequency polygon was used in a study by Williams and Martin (1974), in which the effects of punishment on stuttering behavior was investigated during oral reading adaptation. The following graph (Fig. 8.2) illustrates greater adaptation for the experimental conditions.

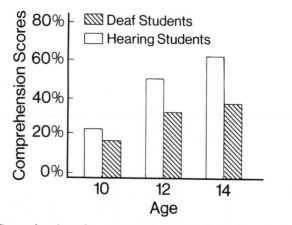

Figure 8.1. Comprehension of occupational concepts for deaf and normal hearing children at three age levels.

Where the frequency polygon is to show both the mean and the standard deviation, vertical bars are shown at each mean to indicate standard deviation. In this type of graph, the horizontal connecting lines are sometimes omitted or, if a trend is to be shown among the standard deviations, connecting lines are added to enclose the entire variance. The following graph (Fig. 8.3) is similar to one presented by Whitehead and Barefoot (1980), in which the oral airflow of deaf and normal speakers was compared. In our simulated graph, it may be seen that the deaf speakers display more variance in airflow than do normal speakers.

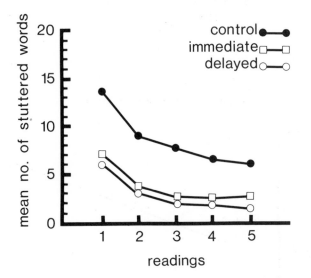

Figure 8.2. Reprinted by permission from Williams, D., and Martin, R., Immediate versus delayed consequences of stuttering responses. J. Speech Hearing Res., 17, 572, 1974.

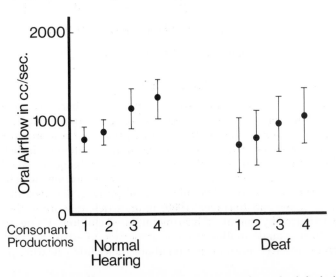

Figure 8.3. Sample frequency polygon for means and standard deviations.

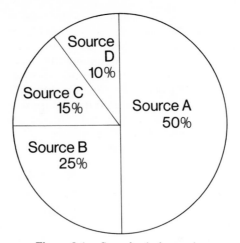

Figure 8.4. Sample circle graph.

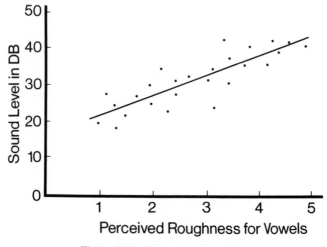

Figure 8.5. Sample scatter plot.

Circle Graphs

The circle graph, more familiarly called a "pie chart" is an effective method for showing how the total sample of a survey is divided into its component proportions. This method of descriptive presentation is used more commonly in business statistics and sociological surveys than in the behavioral sciences. Although it is infrequently used in the speech, language, and hearing area, it is nonetheless a very efficient way to show proportions which add up to 100 % of the total survey. The following graph (Fig. 8.4) uses the format shown by Sweetow and Barrager (1980) in an article describing the quality of care experienced by parents of hearing impaired children. Using simulated data, our chart is made to illustrate the proportion of advisory sources from which parents received misinformation about their child's hearing problem.

The Scatter Plot

This type of presentation is frequently used in experimental phonetics research in which some trends or clusters of data must be illustrated in order to show the spread of individual differences. The following chart (Fig. 8.5) is made to show the kind of data presented by Arnold and Emanuel (1979), in which the perceived vocal roughness was found to be greater in vowels which had higher spectral noise levels. The chart represents hypothetical values from five vowels.

CHAPTER 9 Tests for Differences between Two Groups

t

$$t = \frac{\text{Mean 1} - \text{Mean 2}}{\text{Standard Error of the Difference}}$$

t-TEST FOR INDEPENDENT MEASURES

A test for the difference between two independent groups.

The t-test is probably the most used statistic in the behavioral sciences. It is a ratio which compares the actual difference between two means with the chance difference which could be expected between these means. Chance difference refers to the normal amount of variation which can be found in any set of scores, referred to in this instance as the *standard error of the difference*. If the actual difference between the two means is not much greater than the standard error, it indicates that the differences are literally insignificant, or in other words, not great enough to be "real" differences.

Sample size for the t-test is not critical. However, as the sample size becomes smaller, the assumption that the data are normally distributed becomes much more important to consider. If it becomes obvious that the distributions are widely scattered and irregular, the Mann-Whitney U test would be more appropriate. Slight irregularities in the distribution, however, will not affect the t-test, particularly with larger samples. For this reason it is termed a *robust* statistic. Thirty or more scores is considered a large sample, and seven scores per group is considered small. With the independent t the sample sizes in the two groups need not be equal. *Independent* indicates that the scores do not come from the same group of subjects. A t-test for *dependent* or *related* measures indicates that the two sets of data come from the same subjects, such as hearing thresholds from the same patients, with and without the hearing aid.

In applying the t-test, the null hypothesis states, "There is no difference between the two means." This statistic is used perhaps as often to show that there is no difference as it is to show that a significant difference does exist. For instance, one study (DeHirsch *et al.*, 1964) used the t to show that the vocabularies of prematurely born children were significantly different from those of full-term children. Chaiklin and Ventry (1964), on the other hand used the t to show that there was no difference between mean speech reception thresholds when two different testing methods were used.

Computational Example

Using the study by DeHirsch *et al.* as our computational example, we see that the mean vocabulary for premature children was 181.32 words, while the full-term children had a mean of 224.85 words. The investigators wished to know if this difference was significant. Their sample included fifty-five children in each group. For simplicity our example will substitute very small numbers, for eight mature and seven premature children.

Table 9.1 contains all of the information needed to compute the t-test for independent groups. In computing the t, it is helpful to designate the group with the larger scores as *group 1*, and the smaller scoring group as *group 2*, since the group 2 mean will be subtracted from the group 1 mean.

The next step is to obtain the values called the *sums of squares* for each

Table 9.1. Data for the t-test. Vocabulary scores for mature and premature children.

N	Mature Vocabulary Group 1		Premature Vocabulary Group 2	
	X_1	$X_1{}^2$	X_2	$X_2{}^2$
1	8	64	4	16
2	7	49	5	25
3	6	36	2	4
4	9	81	3	9
5	8	64	6	36
6	7	49	4	16
7	8	64	3	9
8	9	81		

Totals $\sum_1 = 62$ $\sum(X_1{}^2) = 488$ $\sum_2 = 27$ $\sum(X_1{}^2) = 115$
Means $\bar{X}_1 = 7.75$ $\bar{X}_2 = 3.86$
                    $N_1 = 8$ $N_2 = 7$
$(\sum X_1)^2 = 3844$ $(\sum X_2)^2 = 729$

group. These are used in determining the expected difference between the two means, i.e., the *standard error of the mean.*

Mature Group
Sums of Squares, Group₁

$$SS_1 = \sum (x_1{}^2) - \frac{(\sum x_1)^2}{N_1}$$

$$= 488 - \frac{3844}{8}$$

$$= 488 - 480.50$$

$$= 7.50$$

Premature Group
Sums of Squares, Group₂

$$SS_1 = \sum (x_2{}^2) - \frac{(\sum x_2)^2}{N_2}$$

$$= 115 - \frac{729}{7}$$

$$= 115 - 104.14$$

$$= 10.86$$

The standard error of the mean is computed by the pooled variance for the two groups:

Standard Error

$$= \sqrt{\frac{SS_1 + SS_2}{(N_1 + N_2) - 2}\left(\frac{1}{N_1} + \frac{1}{N_2}\right)}$$

$$= \sqrt{\frac{7.50 + 10.86}{(8 + 7) - 2}\left(\frac{1}{8} + \frac{1}{7}\right)}$$

$$= \sqrt{1.41(.268)}$$

$$= \sqrt{.378}$$

$$SE = .615$$

The final step in computation is the *t*-test formula itself. This is to determine whether the difference between means is larger than the standard error. Generally speaking, the difference between the two means should be at least two or three times as large as the standrd error in order to be significant.

$$t = \frac{\bar{x}_1 - \bar{x}_2}{SE} = \frac{\text{Group 1 Mean} - \text{Group 2 Mean}}{\text{Standrd Error of the Mean}}$$

$$= \frac{7.75 - 3.86}{.615}$$

$$= \frac{3.89}{.615}$$

$$= 6.32$$

Significance of the result is determined by looking up the appropriate value in the Table of t (see Appendix H). Values for significance vary according to the degrees of freedom (df) contained in the number of scores used. For the independent t, the df is the total number of scores (15) minus the number of groups (2):

$$df = N_1 + N_2 - 2$$

$$= 8 + 7 - 2$$

$$= 13$$

Our t-test value is 6.32, which is greater than the required value of 3.012 to reject the null hypothesis at the .01 level of confidence, with 13 degrees of freedom. We may conclude (as did DeHirsch *et al.*) that the maturely born children have vocability scores which are significantly greater than those for prematurely born children.

U

$$U = \frac{\text{Proportion of smaller ranks in Group 1}}{\text{Proportion of smaller ranks in Group 2}}$$

MANN-WHITNEY *U* TEST

This is a test of the null hypothesis that there is no difference in the rank order values of the scores found in the two groups of data being compared. In other words, the high ranks and low ranks should be similarly represented in the two groups if the scores were all drawn from the same population, and the groups would not differ significantly. However, if one group is found to contain mostly the lower rank order values, while the other contains higher ranks the groups will be significantly different. Significant difference, therefore, depends upon how little overlap or intermingling of the ranked scores is found across the two groups. The *U* test may be used as a very good alternative to the *t*-test for independent groups; it is not for use with repeated measures. Its *power* (ability to detect significant differences) is about ninety-five percent as effective as the *t*-test unless the sample size is extremely low.

The *U* is preferred over the *t* when the data are not normally distributed, or if the data are already in the form of ranks, as in items arranged according to size or quality. The two groups need not be the same size, and the test is generally used where there are between nine and twenty scores in the larger group, and at least five in the smaller group. Although a few tied scores will not affect the statistic, ties are to be avoided, particularly with smaller samples. When the size of one group is larger than twenty scores, the data tend to be more normally distributed, and a modified computation is used which is based upon the standard error (the *z* score). The *U* may also be used for extremely small samples, such as $N = 3$, for which special tables are available, but the probability levels for samples of less than five scores render the test impractical at that stage. Finally, the *U* test may be used for post hoc analysis, following a significant Kruskal-Wallis *H* test, which is essentially a nonparametric version of the one-way analysis of variance.

Our computational example is based upon a study by Shelton *et al.*, (1965), who employed the Mann-Whitney *U* to test for differences in articulation scores in subjects with two types of palate closure. One group had tight closure, with gaps of less than one millimeter, and the other had gaps greater than one millimeter. Since the articulation scores did not appear to be normally distributed, they were transformed into ranks for treatment with the *U* test. For easier computation in illustrating the *U* test procedure, we will use fictitious articulation scores and smaller groups (Table 9.2).

For computation of the *U*, the actual raw scores are not used; they must first be pooled together and assigned numbers according to rank order. After the ranking procedure, the ranks are then substituted for the original scores, as shown in the example. The ranking procedure is illustrated by the following arrangement (Table 9.3):

It should be noted in this example that there are two scores of 49, which occur at the rank area of 2 and 3. In the case of identical scores, an average rank is assigned, which in this case is 2.5.

Transforming raw scores into ranks is a tedious process, particularly when

89

Table 9.2. Data for the Mann-Whitney U. Articulation scores for two types of palatal closure.

Less than 1 mm. gap	More than 1 mm. gap
76	45
77	49
84	49
85	60
95	64
98	74
	75
	81
	86

Table 9.3. Rank order for raw scores. Articulation scores combined from both groups with assigned ranks.

Scores	Rank
45	1
49	2.5
49	2.5
60	4
64	5
74	6
75	7
76	8
77	9
81	10
84	11
85	12
86	13
95	14
98	15
Combined N = 15	

dealing with a larger number of scores, and it is easy to make an error on this step. A check of ranking errors is recommended, by the formula in which R_1 and R_2 refer to ranks of each of the groups, and N is the total number of pooled scores.

$$\sum R_1 + \sum R_2 = \frac{N(N + 1)}{2}$$

$$69 + 51 = \frac{15(15 + 1)}{2}$$

$$120 = \frac{(15)(16)}{2}$$

$$120 = 120$$

If both sides of the equation are equal, no errors have been made in the ranking process.

The U computation itself is a fairly simple pencil and paper exercise. However, the formula must be used twice—once for each group—in order to

Table 9.4. Computation of the Mann-Whitney U. Ranked data for two types of palatal closure.

Less than 1 mm. Gap		More than 1 mm. Gap	
Score	Rank	Score	Rank
76	8	45	1
77	9	49	2.5
84	11	49	2.5
85	12	60	4
95	14	64	5
98	15	74	6
	69	75	7
		81	10
		86	13
			51
$\sum R_1 = 69$		$\sum R_2 = 51$	
$N_1 = 6$		$N_2 = 9$	

determine which value is smaller. The smaller value, designated as U, is the one to be used for the statistical result. The larger value, designated U', is not used. In our example the U formula for each group is computed by:

Group 1:

$$U = N_1 N_2 + \frac{N_1(N_1 + 1)}{2} - \sum R_1$$

$$= (6)(9) + \frac{6(6 + 1)}{2} - 69$$

$$= 54 + 21 - 69$$

$$= 6$$

Group 2:

$$U = N_1 N_2 + \frac{N_2(N_2 + 1)}{2} - \sum R_2$$

$$= (6)(9) + \frac{(9)(10)}{2} - 51$$

$$= 54 + 45 - 51$$

$$= 48$$

The two U values are 6 and 48. The smaller value, 6, is checked with the table of U to determine whether or not the null hypothesis will be rejected. In the table, the critical value for rejecting the null hypothesis at the .02 level of confidence (two-tailed test) with $N_1 = 6$ and $N_2 = 9$, is a value of 7. Since our value of 6 is smaller than the critical value of 7, the null hypothesis may be rejected. Therefore, the articulation scores for our two groups are found to be significantly different.

U Test for Larger Samples

If there are more than 20 scores in either of the two groups, the data are considered to fall along a somewhat normal distribution, and the z ratio statistic is used. This method involves a bit more computation, and the speed and efficiency of the test becomes somewhat reduced. When using the z test for significance of the U value, the U result from either group may be used, and it is therefore not necessary to compute the U from both groups, as was needed in the small sample method.

To compute the U for larger samples, we shall assume that one group has 21 scores and the other has 10. The U value is computed by the *same formula illustrated previously for small samples*. It makes no difference which of the two groups is used in the formula. Let us say that the result of the U formula gives us a value of $U = 155$. This value is then used to conduct the z test by the following procedure:

$$z = \frac{U - \dfrac{N_1 N_2}{2}}{\sqrt{\dfrac{(N_1)(N_2)(N_1 + N_2 + 1)}{12}}}$$

$$= \frac{155 - \dfrac{(21)(10)}{2}}{\sqrt{\dfrac{(21)(10)(21 + 10 + 1)}{12}}}$$

$$= \frac{50}{\sqrt{\dfrac{6720}{12}}}$$

$$= \frac{50}{23.66}$$

$$= 2.11$$

The table of probability for z indicates that our value of 2.11 exceeds the value 1.96 necessary for significance at the .05 level of confidence. Therefore, the null hypothesis can be rejected, and we may assume that a significant difference exists between the two groups of scores.

Z

$$z = \frac{\text{Proportion from Group 1} - \text{Proportion from Group 2}}{\text{Expected Difference}}$$

PROPORTIONS TEST

A test for the difference between two proportions (or percentages).

A relatively recent addition to the repertoire of familiar statistics is the test for the difference between two proportions. Although this is actually a rather old statistical concept, it has seen little use in the speech and hearing area prior to the current time. Basically, the test implies the use of dichotomous data, in the sense that a trait is counted either present or absent for each individual in order to establish the group proportion. Computation of the z test is relatively simple, although it does require square root. It is most effective when used with larger samples, that is, a combined sample size of thirty or more for both groups, with each group containing at least ten. In evaluating the result, the higher the z value, the more likely the proportions will be significantly different.

In most investigations, the proportions test is not comprehensive enough to answer a research question completely, and it is therefore often used as a secondary statistic in conjunction with some other treatment. This may apply in evaluating the characteristics of various subgroups, such as males and females, smokers and nonsmokers, or large families and small families. The test assumes that the groups are independent, and it can therefore be used with unequal group sizes. However, this feature is not critical to the test results, and it works just as well with related measures. When the result is to show a relationship instead of a simple difference in proportions between two groups, the two-by-two chi square is more suitable for the purpose.

Computational Example

In a study of lipreading perception Wozniak and Jackson (1979) wished to determine whether vowels or diphthongs were the easier to identify. The study included 10 vowels and 6 diphthongs, which were viewed at two different angles (front and side) from the speaker's face. They found that 58% of the vowels were correctly identified and 84% of the diphthongs were correctly identified. The proportions test was to determine whether this difference in proportions was significant.

For our own simplified data, let us say that 10 subjects have tried to perceive a list of syllables accurately by means of lipreading. The 10 vowels and 6 diphthongs have all been presented twice on the list, making a total of 20 vowel syllables and 12 diphthong syllables. The subjects accurately perceived 58% of the vowels and 84% of the diphthongs. For easier computation the group with the larger proportion should be called group 1 and the smaller proportion is called group 2. The data may be summarized as:

Group 1: Total diphthong observations = 12 syllables $\times$ 10 subjects = 120
   = N_1

Total diphthongs correct for all subjects = 101 = X_1

Proportion of diphthongs correct $\dfrac{X_1}{N_1} = \dfrac{101}{120} = .84 = P_1$

93

Group 2: Total vowel observations = 20 syllables × 10 subjects = 200 = N_2

Total vowels correct for all subjects = 116 = X_2

$$\text{Proportion of vowels correct} \frac{X_2}{N_2} = \frac{116}{200} = .58 = P_2$$

To compare the two proportions, the first step is to estimate the total population proportion on the basis of the two samples, or in other words to determine the proportion of correct responses expected simply by drawing a random sample from the whole population.

$$\text{Population proportion} = \frac{X_1 + X_2}{N_1 + N_2}$$

Using the above data from the two groups we have:

$$p = \frac{101 + 116}{120 + 200}$$

$$= \frac{217}{320}$$

$$= .68$$

The p value of .68 is the *weighted mean proportion* from the two samples. To test the significance of the difference between the proportions of correctly perceived vowels (.58) and diphthongs (.84), the p value is now used as part of the z statistic:

$$z = \frac{P_1 - P_2}{\sqrt{\dfrac{p(1-p)}{N_1} + \dfrac{p(1-p)}{N_2}}}$$

$$= \frac{.84 - .58}{\sqrt{\dfrac{(.68)(1-.68)}{120} + \dfrac{(.68)(1-.68)}{200}}}$$

$$= \frac{.26}{\sqrt{\dfrac{.22}{120} + \dfrac{.22}{200}}}$$

$$= \frac{.26}{\sqrt{.002 + .001}}$$

$$= \frac{.26}{.05}$$

$$= 5.20$$

A result which is greater than 1.96 is considered to show differences which are greater than the expected variation, and the proportions of the two groups are therefore significantly different at the .05 level of confidence. For the .01 level of confidence, the z value must exceed 2.58. (Since these criteria apply to all z results, the z table is not always needed.) The 5.20 z value in our computation indicates, in accordance with the results of Wozniak and Jackson, that the proportion of diphthong discrimination (.84) is significantly higher than that for vowels (.58).

t

$$t = \frac{\text{Mean}_1 - \text{Mean}_2}{\text{Standard Error}}$$

t TEST FOR RELATED MEASURES

A test for the difference between two means, from the same group of subjects.

Basically, this is the same t formula as the one previously described, except that when the same subjects are used for both sets of scores the standard error is smaller. As a result, when the same group is used for both sets of scores, smaller differences in the means are apt to be significant. In addition, the degrees of freedom are based upon *pairs* of scores, rather than total scores.

Strictly speaking, the two groups of data need not actually be from the same subjects, but it must be shown that they are somehow correlated. Fundamentally, the statistic is designed to compare pairs of scores across normally distributed groups. This test is often called the t test for repeated measures, but is also known as the dependent t, the t test for correlated observations, or the t test for related measures. It may be used with as few as six pairs of scores, but with fewer pairs the differences must be larger to show significance.

Computational Example

Hearing thresholds for one groups of subjects were tested before and after noise exposure. The t test was used to determine whether or not the change in hearing thresholds was significant (Shearer and Stevens, 1968).

The example consists of pure tone thresholds from 10 subjects obtained before and after a 45 minute exposure to the noise from a power lawn mower. A t-test for repeated measures indicated a significant difference between mean thresholds at the 4000 Hz frequency (Table 9.5).

Table 9.5. Data for the related measures t-test. Hearing thresholds after (X_1) and before (X_2) noise exposure.

Subjects	X_1	X_2	D	D^2
1	5	0	5	25
2	5	0	5	25
3	5	5	0	0
4	0	0	0	0
5	20	10	10	100
6	10	5	5	25
7	30	15	15	225
8	10	0	10	100
9	5	0	5	25
10	5	5	0	0
Totals N = 10	$\sum X_1 = 95$	$\sum X_2 = 40$	$\sum D = 55$	$\sum D^2 = 525$
Means $\bar{X}_1 = 9.5$	$\bar{X}_2 = 4.0$			

$$t = \frac{\bar{X}_1 - \bar{X}_2}{S_{D_{\bar{X}}}}$$

$\bar{X}_1$ = Larger mean score, designated as group 1.

$\bar{X}_2$ = Smaller mean score, designated as group 2.

$S_{D_{\bar{X}}}$ = Expected difference between $\bar{X}_1$ and $\bar{X}_2$.

$$t = \frac{\bar{X}_1 - \bar{X}_2}{\sqrt{\dfrac{\Sigma D^2 - \dfrac{(\Sigma D)^2}{N}}{N(N-1)}}}$$

$$t = \frac{9.5 - 4.0}{\sqrt{\dfrac{525 - \dfrac{(55)^2}{10}}{10(10-1)}}}$$

$$t = \frac{5.5}{\sqrt{2.47}}$$

$$t = \frac{5.5}{1.57}$$

$$t = 3.50$$

The degrees of freedom (*df*) for this formula is the number of *pairs* of scores, minus one. Our example therefore has 9 degrees of freedom, representing a pair of scores for each of the 10 subjects, minus one.

The *t* test result of 3.50 far exceeds the 2.821 value in the *t* table needed to reject the null hypothesis at the .01 level for a one-tailed test. The result therefore indicates a significant difference between means and indicates that a temporary loss in hearing did occur after exposure to lawn mower noise.

T

$$T = \frac{\text{Ranks of} + \text{Changes}}{\text{Ranks of} - \text{Changes}}$$

WILCOXON MATCHED PAIRS TEST

A nonparametric test of the difference between related data groups.

This statistic is based on the assumption that in any retest of the same measures, about half of the scores will show a slight increase and the other half will decrease, on the basis of chance alone. Furthermore, the test assumes that the *amount* of increase and decrease which occurs by chance should be about equal in each direction. The T test, therefore, is to determine how much of a plus or minus difference between two groups of scores will be considered significant. As suggested by the above formula, any change in one direction or the other will produce an uneven numerical balance; since T is based upon the smaller side of the imbalance, very small T values indicate a significant difference.

For practical purposes at least seven pairs should be used in the statistic, although it is possible to test for a difference at .05 with only 6 subjects in a one-tailed test situation. For sample sizes of up to 25 pairs of scores, the table of critical values for T may be used to check for significance of the results. When the sample size exceeds 25 pairs, the z test must be used to determine significance.

As a rule, tied scores are discarded from the data because they contain no information of change either toward plus or minus. If there are quite a large number of ties, however, half can be assigned a plus rank and the other half can be assigned minus ranks of equal value. Since this approach (Hays, 1973) calls for an even number of tied scores, any extra tie should be discarded. This method increases the N slightly, but has no other effect on the statistic. If tied scores are used in this manner, they will all receive the lowest rank, indicating the rank of least change.

The Wilcoxon matched pairs test is frequently discussed in terms of its similarity to the Sign Test, which is also based upon differences in negative and positive scores. The Wilcoxon T, however, utilizes more information than the Sign Test and is therefore a more preferable choice. The T considers not only the direction but also the magnitude of change between the two groups. This lends both *power* and *efficiency* to the test, which means that it readily detects significant diifferences and that it makes maximum use of the available data. For this reason, it represents a good alternative to the t-test for related measures, having about 95% as much power as the t, for use when the data do not appear to be normally distributed. In comparing these two tests, results of the t-test refer to differences in means, whereas the Wilcoxon T implies differences between medians. Since it utilizes ranked data, it may also be used for post hoc analysis following the Friedman Test of rank ordered groups.

Computational Example

In order to test the results of a special type of hearing aid, Harford and Barry (1965) employed the Wilcoxon matched pairs test to compare two sets of speech reception thresholds and two sets of speech discrimination scores. Half of the measures were made without the hearing aid and the other half were made with the hearing aid, using the same 10 subjects for all measures. Their results showed significant improvement both in threshold and discrimination when the CROS hearing aid was worn.

Using our own simplified data to represent discrimination scores for 10 subjects tested with and without the hearing aid, our computation of the Wilcoxon Matched Pairs Test will be (Table 9.6):

Table 9.6. Computation of the Wilcoxon T.

Subjects	Speech Discrimination Scores		Difference	Rank of Difference	Ranks from Less Frequent Signs
	Unaided %	Aided %			
1	92	90	−2	1.5	1.5
2	70	86	+16	3.5	
3	50	68	+18	5	
4	64	80	+16	3.5	
5	90	90	0		
6	56	88	+32	9	
7	86	84	−2	1.5	1.5
8	60	82	+22	6	
9	56	86	+30	8	
10	64	88	+24	7	
				$N = 9$	$= 3 = T$

It should be noted that $N = 9$; there are only nine ranked differences, since subject number 5 did not show a difference in scores and was omitted from the computation. The minus sign appears less frequently than the plus sign, so our $T = 3$ is based upon the total ranks for the differences in the minus direction. The T value of 3 (the value of the less frequent sign) is checked for significance by using the table of critical values for the Wilcoxon Matched Pairs Test, under the heading of $N = 9$, for a one tailed test. Since we knew before the experiment that subjects tend to hear somewhat better with hearing aids, the test was to see whether this difference would be significant or not, and a one-tailed test would therefore be appropriate. (If there were no reason to know which direction the change would take, a two-tailed test would be used in considering the probability of the result.) The table of T values indicates that a T of 3 or less is required to reject the null hypothesis at the .01 level for a one tailed test. Therefore, we may assume that the discrimination scores are significantly improved when the subjects are wearing this type of hearing aid.

THE WILCOXON T FOR LARGE SAMPLES

When 25 or more pairs of scores are used in the sample, the data are considered to fall into a fairly normal distribution, and the significance of the result may be derived from a z test. That is, the difference between the two groups may be judged as to whether or not both groups are likely to fall under the same normal curve. If one group is found to be too near the outer boundary of the curve (i.e., the tail), it is considered to belong to a different population, and the difference is therefore significant.

Computational Example

For our example we shall consider a study by Hudgins and Cullinan (1978) in which 40 students repeated a series of test sentences containing several types of sentence structure. Results were scored on the basis of sentence error in the repetition, and latency of response. Both short and long sentences were used for each structural type. The investigators wished to know whether the type of sentence structure influenced the imitative errors and response latency of the student repetitions of the sentences. Since the intersubject data varied in a wide and somewhat irregular fashion, the Wilcoxon Matched Pairs T test was used in the statistical treatment.

While the study itself considered many combinations of comparison in comprehensive detail, our computational example will use simplified data to represent only one aspect of the original study. Hypothetical scores representing the repetition errors from 25 students for the subject-focus vs. the object-focus types of sentences are displayed in Table 9.7.

Table 9.7. T computation for larger samples. Errors made by 25 students during elicited imitation responses for subject-focus and object-focus types of sentences.

| Subjects | Errors | | Difference | Rank of Difference | Ranks of Less Frequent Sign |
	Subject-focus	Object-focus			
1	5	3	−2	9.5	9.5
2	2	3	1	4	
3	6	9	3	14.5	
4	4	1	−3	14.5	14.5
5	2	6	4	18.5	
6	8	4	−4	18.5	18.5
7	7	8	1	4	
8	2	8	6	23.5	
9	4	5	1	4	
10	3	8	5	21	
11	8	5	−3	14.5	14.5
12	6	7	1	4	
13	4	3	−1	4	4
14	1	6	5	21	
15	3	5	2	9.5	
16	3	4	1	4	
17	5	3	−2	9.5	9.5
18	6	9	3	14.5	
19	2	4	2	9.5	
20	9	8	−1	4	4
21	3	9	6	23.5	
22	1	4	3	14.5	
23	1	8	7	25	
24	6	9	3	14.5	
25	2	7	5	21	
26	1	9	8	26	

$$T = 74.5$$
$$N = 26$$

Computation of the Wilcoxon Matched Pairs Test for large samples:

$$z = \frac{T - \dfrac{N(N + 1)}{4}}{\sqrt{\dfrac{N(N + 1)(2N + 1)}{24}}}$$

$$= \frac{74.5 - \dfrac{26(26 + 1)}{4}}{\sqrt{\dfrac{26(26 + 1)(52 + 1)}{24}}}$$

$$= \frac{- 101}{\sqrt{\dfrac{37206}{24}}}$$

$$= 2.56$$

In checking the probability level of the z result, the criterion for significance at .05 is a value of 1.96, the .02 level is a value of 2.33, and .01 requires a value of 2.58. With these basic criteria values in mind, it is not necessary to refer to a z table in establishing significance of the result. Since our z result of 2.56 exceeds the criterion of 2.33, it is determined that the two groups are significantly different at the .02 level of confidence (for a two-tailed test). In referring to our original example, our simulated data are found to display a significantly greater number of errors on the subject-focus sentences than on the self-focus sentences, as concluded in the Hudgins and Cullinan study.

Z

$$z = \frac{+ \text{ Changes}}{- \text{ Changes}} = \frac{.50}{.50}$$

SIGN TEST

A nonparametric test for plus or minus change in related measures.

As illustrated in the above formula, the Sign Test is a very simple statistic which assumes that when anything is remeasured, half of the new measures will naturally be slightly larger and half will be slightly smaller than the original measures. It is an easily computed statistic which is particularly useful when the direction of any change is the only information to be considered, as in clinical situations where the new condition might be judged only as "better" or "worse." The *amount* of change is not considered in these measures, either because it can not be estimated accurately or because it is simply not in the test situation, as in success vs. failure. Results of the Sign Test indicate whether or not an apparent change is actually significant.

The Sign Test is essentially a repeated-measures statistic, but is also appropriate for matched groups in which the measures are made on equivalent but not identical subjects, as in paired experimental vs. control groups. It is more effectively used with data involving 10 to 25 pairs of scores, although it is possible to show significance with as few as six pairs if large differences are apparent. If there is no difference between a pair of observations (tied scores), that pair should be discarded. As sample size becomes larger, statistics generally tend to increase in power, but this does not hold true for the Sign Test. For sample sizes of 30 or more pairs, the Sign Test becomes only about 65% as powerful as alternative tests. Its main weakness is that if there are large differences between the pairs of scores, this information is not taken into account in calculating significance and there is a chance of overlooking some significant differences which might be present. When a significant difference is not detected by a statistic, it is called a *Type II Error*. If the relative magnitude of the difference between pairs can be estimated, the Wilcoxon Matched Pairs *T*, rather than the Sign Test, should be used because of its greater power to detect significance. When both groups of scores are normally distributed, the *t*-test for related measures is of course preferred.

Computational Example

Silverman (1976) used two equivalent groups of students to rate a speech sample containing lateral lisps, as compared with a sample containing only normal speech. Ratings were made on a seven-point scale which used a number of descriptive categories to evaluate the two speech samples. The ratings for lisping were compared with ratings for normal speakers, and assigned a plus or minus according to the direction in which the ratings changed.

For our computation we shall use only nine pairs of ratings, in which one pair of ratings was the same for both speakers (Table 9.8). When the tied

Table 9.8. Summary of data for the sign test.

Number of Paired Scores	Mean Ratings of Speech Samples		Direction of Difference
	Normal Speech	Lisping Speech	
1	6	4	−
2	6	5	−
3	5	4	−
4	7	6	−
5	3	4	+
6	6	3	−
7	6	2	−
8	5	4	−
9 (omit)	5	5	0
		Number of fewer signs = 1	

scores are discarded we have an N of only eight pairs. Since our N is less than 10 pairs, we shall use the .05 level of confidence instead of the .01. With a larger N, rejection of the null hypothesis at .01 would be more feasible.

$$z = \frac{(\text{number of pairs})(.5) - \text{number of fewer signs}}{\sqrt{(\text{number of pairs})(.5)(.5)}}$$

$$= \frac{(8)(.5) - 1}{\sqrt{(8)(.5)(.5)}}$$

$$= \frac{4 - 1}{\sqrt{2}}$$

$$= \frac{3}{1.41}$$

$$= 2.13$$

The z value must be at least 1.96 in order to show a significant difference at .05. This probability value is based on the idea that the change could go in either direction: a two-tailed test. Since z probability does not utilize degrees of freedom, the same values apply to all z computations, and the use of a table is therefore unnecessary. Regardless of the sample size, the 1.96 value is the criterion for significance at .05, and the value of 2.58 is the criterion for the .01 level of confidence. Our z of 2.13 exceeds the 1.96 necessary for significances at .05.

As in Silverman's study, our hypothetical data indicate that judgments toward lateral lispers are significantly less favorable than are judgments of normal speakers. The study concluded, on the basis of these judgments, that the lateral lisp constitutes a serious speech defect and should be treated in the schools as early as possible.

Z

Estimated Proportion = Observed Proportion

BINOMIAL TEST

Although not widely used, the Binomial Test is very helpful for the specialized situation where all subjects or all scores fall in to one of two distinct categories. For instance, the subjects may be composed of males and females, or the scores may be classified as pass or fail. The Binomial Test is to let us know if the observed proportion of any two dependent categories is different from the proportion estimated by chance. By *dependent categories* we mean that the two proportions must equal 100%, or in other words the total group. This, if 40% of one group are males, we know that the other 60% has to be females, or if 55% of a group heard better in the right ear, the remaining 45% must have heard better in the left ear. All test scores to be evaluated by this statistical treatment must be forced into two categories; there is no provision for any other classification of the results.

In the type of data to be used and in the nature of its results, the Binomial Test closely resembles other tests which deal with binomial information, such as the Chi Square, the Proportions Test, and the Sign Test. The Binomial Test, however, is an exceptionally convenient and very simply computed technique for use where either the subjects or the test stimuli are set up in two equally matched groups, where the probability is that the two groups should score the same. The estimated results in these cases is a 50–50 distribution; i.e., half of those who pass a test should be from group 1 and the other half should be from group 2. It should be noted, however, that the Binomial Test may be used with any two proportions which add up to 100%; the situation where both groups are of equal size is quite common and is the simplest to compute.

Research projects which deal with articulation development and language development are particularly well suited for use of the Binomial Test because they characteristically involve equally matched groups, such as male-female, Black-Caucasian, rural-urban, lower socio-economic level-middle level, language delayed-nondelayed, etc. The null hypothesis in these studies usually states that there is "no difference in performance between the two groups", and the Binomial Test can easily determine whether this null hypothesis should be rejected.

The power and efficiency of the Binomial Test seems to be as good as that of any of the other binomial techniques, which means that if continuous data are forced into a binomial classification (high scores vs. low scores), this test will not be quite as sensitive as the t-test or other parametric methods. However, as Siegel (1956) points out, if the data are inherently binomial, this test is as effective as anything else which might be used.

Computational Example

In a study to evaluate the ability of deaf subjects to recognize words tactually through skin vibration, Oller, *et al.* (1980) presented a list of words through a vibrating device on the forearms of the subjects. At each presentation the subject indicated which of two words shown on a card was felt on the arm. Since each choice allowed an equal chance of being right or wrong, we can assume that the probability for the test was 50% correct and 50% incorrect, which could be achieved by guessing at all presentations. The investigators wished to find whether certain types of words scored better than 50% chance response. Each word was presented 20 times in the total series and each subject was evaluated individually. By chance alone, each subject would therefore make 10 correct choices and 10 incorrect choices.

If we assume that a subject scored 16 correct choices out of 20 presentations, the critical question is, "Is 16 out of 20 significantly better than chance?" The *simplified z formula*, which is designed in this case to apply *only when the chance probability is 50%*, appears as:

$$z = \frac{\text{Number correct} - \dfrac{\text{Total number of choices}}{2}}{\sqrt{\dfrac{\text{Total number of choices}}{4}}}$$

Using our hypothetical subject's score of 16 correct out of 20 presentations, the numerical example is:

$$z = \frac{16 - \dfrac{20}{2}}{\sqrt{\dfrac{20}{4}}}$$

$$= 2.67$$

The z value may be easily checked without referring to a table, since 1.96 always has significance at p. $< .05$ and 2.58 has p. $< .01$. The present z value of 2.67 exceeds 2.58 and is therefore significant at better than the .01 level of confidence. We may assume from the result of the Binomial Test that the word discrimination score of 16 is significantly better than chance, and that the subject was able to receive accurate verbal cues by tactile stimulation.

CHAPTER 10 Tests for Differences among Several Groups with One Variable

F

$$F = \frac{\text{Variance between groups}}{\text{Variance within population}}$$

ANALYSIS OF VARIANCE:

General Description

It may be convenient to think of the analysis of variance (AOV) as being very much like the t-test in that it tests for differences between groups of scores and is based upon normally distributed data. The essential difference is that it considers the variances rather than the means as the basic factor in comparing groups of scores. The null hypothesis then assumes that all scores are taken from the same population and that all variances are a part of one big variance from that population. Since we are more accustomed to thinking about comparing means rather than variances, this summary statement will be helpful in comprehending the logic of the analysis of variance: *If the groups of scores are normally distributed and have the same variances, they will also have the same means.* Therefore, although we are not actually comparing mean scores, our results will be the same as though we were. Comparing variances by this method is simply an indirect way of comparing means.

As we have shown in the preceding discussion of the test, it must be assumed that the scores within each group are normally distributed before the data can be treated effectively with an analysis of variance. Although this assumption is critical to the analysis, it is not particularly restrictive, since most data samples in the behavioral sciences naturally tend to fall into a normal distribution pattern. Furthermore, the robust nature of the AOV allows for minor deviations in the variance pattern. Therefore, unless the data are based upon ranked scores, percentages, small Ns or obviously skewed information, the chances are that the distribution will fall into a fairly normal pattern. As a general rule, 30 or more scores will tend to normalize the distribution.

As with many other statistical formulas, the analysis of variance indicates whether or not there is really a difference between groups of scores. The observed diference is compared with a difference which could be obtained by chance. (Chance differences are usually due to minor variations in the sensitivity of the subjects, the experimenters, or the measuring instruments.) If the observed difference is about the same as the chance difference, we conclude that the observed difference was probably just a random occurrence, which of course would not be significant.

The basic formula, as shown in the beginning of this section, is

$$F = \frac{\text{Variance between groups}}{\text{Variance within population}}$$

The actual computation, however, is usually depicted by

$$F = \frac{SS_{\text{between groups}}}{SS_{\text{within groups}}}$$

The *SS* notation indicates *sums of squares*. During the computation, this term should not be confused with the summation of the squared scores, which is merely a preliminary part of the mathematical procedure. Sums of squares refers to the sums of the squared deviations around the mean, or in other words, the variance. Two other terms should also be mentioned at this point in order to avoid later confusion. These are called the *residual* and the *error term*. Very briefly, these two terms refer to the population variance, and are used in computation of the denominator of the F formula for some types of the basic AOV treatment method.

In the computation of a relatively complex analysis of variance, it is quite easy to make serious mathematical errors. Such errors usually appear in the form of a negative value in one or more sums of squares. Since this part of the AOV computation is derived from the average variance of scores around the mean, *there is no such thing as a negative sum of squares*. The elusiveness of this type of error is notorious, to the point where it is sometimes necessary to call upon someone else to check the computation from a fresh point of view. When a negative sum of squares appears, a likely source of error is in any of the computational steps where the numbers seem to be extraordinarily large, for this is a common symptom of miscalculation in the analysis of variance.

F

ONE-WAY ANALYSIS OF VARIANCE

A test for differences among three or more independent groups.

This statistical treatment method is the simplest of the analysis of variance techniques. It may be viewed as an expanded version of the t-test for independent measures, for use with three or more groups.

As an illustration, we will consider a study of language development in which six age groups were given a test for comprehension of pronouns (Bountress, 1978). Eight children from each age group were tested, and a general trend of improvement with age seemed to be evident. An analysis of variance was used to determine whether the differences between age groups were significant. Since different subjects were used in each test group, the results were computed by a one-way analysis. (If a sequence of tests were performed on the *same subjects* over a period of time, a treatments-by-subjects analysis would be used.) On the basis of the results, Bountress reported a significant difference in pronoun comprehension among the age groups.

Computational Example

In a simplified version of the analysis, our own scores will be used to represent test data for five subjects from each of three age groups.

Sums of Squares Between Groups $= SS_{between}$

$$SS_{between} = \frac{(each\ sum)^2}{Subjects\ per\ group} - \frac{(Grand\ Total)^2}{Total\ Subjects}$$

$$= \frac{(17)^2 + (36)^2 + (39)^2}{5} - \frac{(92)^2}{15}$$

$$= \frac{289 + 1296 + 1521}{5} - \frac{8464}{15}$$

$$= \frac{3106}{5} - 564.27$$

$$= 56.93$$

Sums of Squares Within Groups $= SS_{within}$

$$SS_{within} = Each\ \chi^2 - \frac{(Each\ sum)^2}{Group\ Subjects}$$

$$= 644 - \frac{(17)^2 + (36)^2 + (39)^2}{5}$$

$$= 644 - \frac{289 + 1296 + 1521}{5}$$

$$= 644 - 621.2$$

$$= 22.80$$

Degrees of Freedom $= df$

$df_{total} = N - 1 = 15 - 1 = 14$
$df_{between} = \text{Groups} - 1 = 3 - 1 = 2$
$df_{within} = (\text{Subjects per group})(\text{Groups}) - \text{Groups} = (5)(3) - 3 = 15 - 3 = 12$

Computation of the F ratio

Source of Variation	df	Sum of Squares	Mean Squares*	F
$SS_{between}$	2	56.93	28.46	14.98
SS_{within}	12	22.80	1.90	

$$F = \frac{\text{Mean Squares Between}}{\text{Mean Squares Within}} = \frac{28.47}{1.90} = 14.98$$

$$* \text{ Mean Squares} = \frac{\text{Sum of Squares}}{\text{Degrees of Freedom}}$$

The F result in our example ($F = 14.98$) exceeds considerably the F table value of 6.93 necessary for significance at .01, with 2 and 12 degrees of freedom. This indicates that there is a significant difference among the pronoun comprehension scores of the age groups in our example, analogous to the study reported by Bountress.

Our F result tells us only that a difference exists among the three groups, but does not indicate exactly which or how many groups differ. Visual inspection of the means (age 4 = 3.40; age 6 = 7.20; age 8 = 7.80) suggests that age 4 is probably different from ages 6 and 8, and that ages 6 and 8 are about the same. In many studies, this analysis of the results is sufficient, and no further statistical treatment is necessary. Let us say, however, that the various group differences in this case are important for our conclusion. We must therefore pursue the result further by what is called post hoc analysis.

Post hoc analysis is a procedure which can be used following a significant F result in the analysis of variance. Its purpose is to specify which of the possible comparisons accounted for significance in the F ratio. When the F score is

Table 10.1. Data for the one-way analysis of variance. Pronoun comprehension scores for 15 subjects representing three age groups.

			Ages			
	4		6		8	
	X	X²	X	X²	X	X²
	2	4	5	25	8	64	N = 15
	3	9	8	64	7	49	Groups = 5
	5	25	9	81	9	81	Subjects per group = 5
	3	9	8	64	6	36	
	4	16	6	36	9	81	
Totals $\sum X$	17		36		39		=92
$\sum (X^2)$		63		270		311	= 644
Means $\bar{X}$	3.40		7.20		7.80		= 6.13 = Grand Mean

not significant, there is of course no point in applying post hoc analysis because it has already been shown that none of the comparisons are significant. As an illustration of post hoc analysis, computation of the Tukey Test using the present F test data is shown in the section entitled *Transformations and Post Hoc Analysis* for the Analysis of Variance.

H

Σ Group 1 Ranks = Σ Group 2 Ranks, etc.

KRUSKAL-WALLIS H TEST

A nonparametric test for differences among three or more independent groups.

The rationale of the Kruskal-Wallis H test is that if all scores are assembled into one large group, assigned to rank order, and dropped into several piles, the ranks in each pile will add up about to the same value. The basic design for this test is the same as that for the single-factor analysis of variance, described earlier. The main assumptions are (1) that different subjects are used for each condition, and (2) that the data may be arranged in rank order. Since H test results are checked for significance on a table of Chi Square, at least five subjects should be included in each category of treatment. It is not necessary to have the same number of subjects in each category.

Computational Example

The first step is to arrange the scores from all categories into a single rank order. The following table presents data similar to that obtained by Costello and Schoen (1978), who studied the results from three types of therapy approaches to the correction of frontal lisp. The three methods were videotape, audiotape, and live. The videotape and audiotape programs were administered by trained paraprofessionals and the live presentation was conducted by a professional speech clinician. The investigators wished to determine whether a significant difference appeared in the results achieved from the three methods, in order to assess the effectiveness of the paraprofessionals.

In the following table, each score has been replaced with a ranking number, with the smallest score receiving a rank of 1.

Note: The values 12 and 3 are constants in the H formula.

$$H = \left(\frac{12}{(\text{Subjects})(\text{Subjects} + 1)} \right) \left(\frac{(\text{Each Total})^2}{\text{Each \# Subjects}} \right) - 3(\text{Subjects} + 1)$$

$$= \left(\frac{12}{(15)(16)} \right) \left(\frac{1764}{5} + \frac{1024}{5} + \frac{2116}{5} \right) - (3)(16)$$

$$= \frac{12}{240} (352.8 + 204.8 + 423.2) - 48$$

$$= .05 \ (980.8) - 48$$

$$= 49.04 - 48$$

$$= 1.04$$

The results of the H test are interpreted from a table of Chi Square, with the degrees of freedom determined by conditions-minus-one ($df = 3 - 1 = 2$). Since the present H value of 1.04 is considerably less than the Chi Square

Table 10.2. Data for the Kruskal-Wallis H Test. Rank order of achievement for 15 children, divided into three therapy groups.

	Videotape	Audiotape	Live
	1	11	5
	7	2	8
	9	3	6
	10	4	14
	15	12	13
$\sum$ Ranks	42	32	46
(Ranks)^2	1764	1024	2116

value of 5.99 necessary for the .05 level of confidence, the hypothesis of no difference among the three articulation groups is maintained. Therefore, as noted in the report of Costello and Schoen, the three methods of therapy are equally effective.

$$\chi^2$$

$$\chi^2 = \frac{(\text{observed frequency} - \text{expected frequency})^2}{\text{expected frequency}}$$

CHI SQUARE

A test for differences among several multiple choice categories.

The Chi Square test is used primarily for a binomial type of data or in cases where the variables can be classified according to broad categories, such as "yes vs. no," "young vs. old," "high vs. low," etc. It may also be used for data which is in the nature of a multiple-choice decision, where each subject is asked to pick only one of several possible categories. It is considered to be a nonparametric statistic, since it does not compare means. When the data are normally distributed and need not be treated as binomial, a comparison of means (i.e., t-test or F test) is a more sensitive treatment, and therefore preferable to the Chi Square.

Where the Chi Square is to be used to evaluate several related variables it is simpler to break the data down into separate Chi Square tests, rather than to attempt to combine several variables into one large block, as is typically performed in the analysis of variance. Data for this test should be sufficient to allow an expected frequency of at least 5 per cell in order to give the statistic acceptable stability. Less than five puts to much weight upon any single observation.

Computational Example

Perhaps the simplest type of Chi Square design is one in which *each subject is asked to make one multiple-choice judgement.* For example, in order to determine which type of stuttering block is judged to be "most severe," four speakers were trained to stutter on the same number of words, with each speaker using a different type of block (Williams, 1980). Recorded samples were played to 20 listeners, and each listener was asked to select "the most severe stutterer." The following results were obtained:

In the present example, 20 listeners were chosen, so as to allow an expected frequency of 5 for each of the four cells, assuming that all stutterers are equally severe. The computational table is arranged according to the formula $\chi^2 = \Sigma \frac{(fo - fe)^2}{fe}$.

The significance of the result is determined in the table of Chi Square

Table 10.3. Computation of the chi square.

Type of block	Observed frequency fo	Expected frequency fe	fo−fe	(fo−fe)²	$\frac{(fo - fe)^2}{fe}$
Prolongations	1	5	−4	16	3.2
Repetitions	6	5	1	1	.2
Silent Pause	3	5	−2	4	.8
Audible Pause	10	5	5	25	5.0
	20	20			$\chi^2 = 9.2$

according to the appropriate degrees of freedom. In this case there are three degrees of freedom (df = categories − 1). Table 10.3 indicates that the value must exceed 7.815 before the null hypothesis of "no difference from the expected frequency" can be rejected at the .05 confidence level. Our value of 9.2 indicates that the observed frequencies do vary significantly from the expected frequency of 5, and that the null hypothesis is therefore rejected. Inspection of the data indicates that blocks having audible pauses were most often judged as the most severe form of stuttering.

F

$$F = \frac{\text{Variance between groups}}{\text{Variance within combined groups,}}$$
called the "residual" term

TREATMENTS-BY-SUBJECTS ANALYSIS OF VARIANCE

A test for difference among several groups having normal distribution. One group of subjects takes all tests (treatments).

Treatments should be counterbalanced to eliminate serial effects, unless it is used as a test for trend.

The F result from this statistic will answer the question: Is there a difference among the treatment scores?

The treatments-by-subjects analysis of variance is essentially an expansion of the t-test for related measures. From another viewpoint it is the related measures version of the one-way AOV. The main criterion is that *all subjects take all tests*.

This statistic has wide usage in the speech, language, and hearing areas because of the relatively small number of subjects available in clinical populations. This is in contrast to experimental psychology, which draws large numbers of subjects from undergraduate classes, and therefore is inclined to use different subjects for each type of treatment. The $T \times S$ design is also known as a single factor analysis with repeated measures. The difference between the subjects themselves is usually not of interest in the results.

The mechanics of this method are basically to see whether the variation among treatment scores is bigger than the variance among subject's scores. If the difference between the treatments is no bigger than the variation among subjects as a whole it means that the differences are unimportant, or in other words "not significant."

The treatments-by-subjects design has many advantages. Since each subject takes all tests, there is no problem concerning selection of homogeneous groups of subjects for each test. In order to avoid the serial order effect on consecutive tests, these are usually counterbalanced, which reduce the learning effect and similar influences which may occur from one treatment to the next. However, in clinical studies which test for periodic progress, the succession of tests is an important aspect of the results, i.e., testing for a significant trend.

In summary, the test calls for considerably fewer subjects than that used in

Figure 10.1. Data sheet for the $T \times S$ design.

Subjects	Treatment 1	Treatment 2	Treatment 3
1			
2			
3			
4			
5			
—			

a randomized design, it has the benefit of using each subject as its own control, and the repeated measures feature of the design is well-suited to periodic tests of clinical progress.

Computational Example

The example is drawn from a study which compared three methods of sampling articulation performance in children (DuBois and Bernthal, 1978). The investigators wished to compare test scores from continuous speech, modeled continuous speech, and spontaneous speech-naming tasks, using a group of 18 young children. For simplicity our hypothetical scores will represent only five children tested by the three methods.

Sums of Squares Between Treatments $= SS_{treatments}$

$$SS_{treatments} = \frac{\text{Each Total Squared}}{\text{Subjects}} - \frac{(\text{Grand Total})^2}{(\text{Treatments})(\text{Subjects})}$$

$$SS_{treatments} = \frac{(17)^2 + (38)^2 + (52)^2}{5} - \frac{(107)^2}{(3)(5)}$$

$$= \frac{289 + 1444 + 2704}{5} - \frac{11449}{15}$$

$$= 887.40 - 763.27$$

$$= 124.13$$

Residual Sums of Squares $= SS_{residual}$
Note: Residual Sums of Squares is the error term in this analysis.

$$SS_{residual} = \text{Total Squared Scores} - \frac{\text{Each Total Squared}}{\text{Subjects}}$$
$$- \frac{\text{Each Subject Total Squared}}{\text{Treatments}} + \frac{(\text{Grand Total})^2}{(\text{Treatments})(\text{Subjects})}$$

Table 10.4. Computation of the treatments-by-subjects AOV articulation scores from three test methods.

Subjects	Continuous Speech		Modeled Continuous speech		Spontaneous Picture Naming		Subject Totals	
	X	X²	X	X²	X	X²	Σ	Σ²
1	2	4	6	36	9	81	17	289
2	5	25	9	81	11	121	25	625
3	4	16	8	64	10	100	22	484
4	3	9	8	64	10	100	21	441
5	3	9	7	49	12	144	22	484

Totals: ΣX 17   38   52   = 107 Grand Total
Totals: ΣX^2 63   294   546 = 903 Grand Total Squares

Means: $\bar{X}$ 3.40   7.60   10.40
Number of Subjects = N = 5
Number of Treatments = 3

ΣX = Sum of Raw Scores
ΣX^2 = Each score is squared and the values are summed.
$\bar{X}$ = Mean = average score

Table 10.5 Results of the T × S analysis of variance.

Source of Variation	SS	df	MS	F
Treatments	124.13	2	62.06	110.82
Residual	4.53	8	.56	

$$= \quad 903 - \frac{(17)^2 + (38)^2 + (52)^2}{5}$$

$$- \frac{289 + 625 + 484 + 441 + 484}{3} + \frac{(107)^2}{(3)(5)}$$

$$= \quad 903 - \frac{4437}{5} - \frac{2323}{3} + \frac{11449}{15}$$

$$= \quad 4.54$$

Degrees of Freedom = df

$df_{\text{treatments}} = \text{Treatments} - 1 = 3 - 1 = 2$

$df_{\text{residual}} = (\text{subjects} - 1)(\text{treatments} - 1) = (4)(2) = 8$

$$\text{Mean Squares} = \frac{SS}{df} = MS$$

Computation of the *F* Ratio:

$$F = \frac{MS_{\text{treatments}}}{MS_{\text{residual}}} = \frac{62.06}{.56}$$

In the table of *F* distribution, using 2 *df* for the numerator and 8 *df* for the denominator we find that a value of 8.65 is necessary for a significant difference at the .01 level of confidence. The present *F* ratio of 110.82 far exceeds the necessary minimum value, indicating a highly significant *F* result.

On the basis of our *F* result we may assume with 99 percent certainty that the articulation test methods produce significantly different mean scores. Inspection of the means for the three articulation test methods reveals that the greatest difference appears between Continuous Speech (mean = 3.40) and Spontaneous Picture Naming (mean = 10.40). In the light of a significant *F* result it can be assumed that the largest difference is significant, but the significance of the other group differences is still uncertain at this point. (Purely on the basis of statistical probability, however, it is *possible* to derive a significant *F* in which none of the group differences are significant, but this is a rare anomaly which need not be considered on a practical basis.)

If it is important for the investigator to point out all of the differences among the various treatment groups, their significance may be tested by *post hoc* methods described in the section following the analysis of variance examples.

Q

Q: Proportion 1 = Proportion 2 = Proportion 3

COCHRAN Q TEST

A non parametric test for difference among related groups of binomial data.

This test is primarily intended for pass-fail data in a situation where one group of subjects is tested under several conditions. Since the pass-fail criterion is used for many screening test procedures, such as hearing, language, and articulation screening of school children, the Q test would appear well-suited for research in these topics. As shown in the conceptual formula at the beginning of the section, the statistic is based upon the null hypothesis that the proportion of pass vs. fail (or yes vs. no) will not vary from one group to the next. In this respect, it is an expansion of the Proportions Test, to be used with three or more proportions instead of two. Since it is a comparison test for several related groups, its experimental design is essentially the same as the treatments-by-subjects analysis of variance.

It is not recommended for very small samples, because the result of the test is evaluated as a Chi Square distribution. Ten or more subjects are suggested. The concept of "power" can not be established very well by comparing the Q test results with those from other statistics, because when other types of data are forced into a binomial distribution, some of the information is lost. The test, therefore, can only be considered applicable to pass-fail information, and is not actually an alternative to the normally distributed treatments-by-subjects AOV or the Friedman Test for ranked data.

Computational Example

One aspect of an investigation into the effectiveness of testing procedures for nonorganic hearing loss was to compare the results of four tests used on the same group of subjects (Monroe and Martin, 1977). Since this type of test is scored on a pass-fail basis, Cochran's Q test was used for the comparison.

Fictitious data representing the scores of 10 subjects on four tests is shown in the Table 10.6:

Note: Although the Cochran Q test is relatively simple to compute, special attention should be paid to the parentheses and brackets, which represent a particular hazard for errors.

$$Q = \frac{(\text{treatments} - 1)\left[(\text{treatments})(\text{each treatment squared}) - \left(\frac{\text{Grand}}{\text{Total}}\right)^2\right]}{(\text{treatments})(\text{Grand Total}) - \sum \text{each subject squared}}$$

$$= \frac{(4 - 1)[(4)(178) - (24)^2]}{(4)(24) - 64}$$

$$= \frac{408}{32}$$

$$= 12.75$$

Table 10.6. Data for the Cochran Q test. Pass-fail results from ten subjects with feigned hearing loss on four tests.

Subjects	Speech-Pure Tone Difference	Ascending-Descending Thresholds	Pure Tone Stenger Test	Pure Tone DAF	Σ	Σ^2
1	+	−	−	+	2	4
2	+	+	−	−	2	4
3	+	+	−	+	1	1
4	+	+	−	−	2	4
5	+	+	−	−	2	4
6	+	−	−	−	3	9
7	+	−	−	+	2	4
8	+	−	−	−	3	9
9	−	+	−	−	3	9
10	−	−	−	−	4	16

Minus Scores	=	2	5	10	7	= 24
Totals Squared	=	4	25	100	49	178 64
Treatments	=	4				
Grand Total	=	24				
Σ (each treatment squared) = 178						
Σ (each Subject Squared) = 64						

Degrees of Freedom (df) = Treatments − 1 = 4 − 1 = 3

The significance of the Q test result is determined through the table of chi square values. With 3 degrees of freedom, the Q result of 12.75 exceeds the chi square value of 11.34 at the .01 level of confidence, indicating a significant difference among the hearing test methods. Inspection of the data chart indicates that the best record was achieved by the Pure Tone Stenger Test.

$$\chi^2$$

χ^2: Group 1 Ranks = Group 2 Ranks = Group 3 Ranks

FRIEDMAN'S TEST

A test for difference among several rank-ordered groups, using related measure.

This test is essentially a treatments-by-subjects design for use with data which are in rank-order form or which do not appear to have a normal distribution. It is a test which employs related measures, or in other words, all measures come from the same subjects. This method is particularly suited to the situation where several conditions are rated as being higher or lower than the others, with no need to indicate *how much* higher or lower. In some instances, the judges are simply asked to put the examples in rank order from highest to lowest; in other instances, a set of raw scores may be transformed into rank order.

Friedman's Test may be used with as few as three treatments and three subjects, employing tables of exact probabilities. However, with so few items, the ranks must be stacked perfectly in order to obtain the .05 level of significance. The test is more practical when there are at least four treatments, with at least five subjects. Fifteen or more subjects would be considered a large sample. Where there are obvious reservations about the normal distribution of data, Friedman's test is considered to be a good substitute for the treatments-by-subjects analysis of variance, and is generally more powerful than the Cochran Q test (Siegel, 1956).

Computational Example

In the example to be computed, Healey *et al.*, (1976) observed stutterers' frequency of nonfluencies during four types of verbal production. Eight stutterers read familiar and unfamiliar material to produce singing and oral reading. The investigators wished to know whether there was a difference in relative fluency among the four conditions.

For our simplified example we shall make up data for six stutterers producing the four types of performance described by Healey *et al.*

Relative fluency for each vocalization condition is first ranked according to amount of stuttering. By this technique, differences among the basic fluency of the stutterers do not play an important role in the results. The important part of the data is simply whether he was "better" or "worse" in comparing one condition with another. Least stuttering receives a rank of "1" and most stuttering receives a rank of "4".

Sums of Squares for Treatments = $SS_{treatments}$

$$SS_{treatments} = \frac{\sum (\text{Each Sum}^2)}{\text{Subjects}} - \frac{(\text{Grand Total})^2}{(\text{Subjects})(\text{Treatments})}$$

$$= \frac{361 + 64 + 484 + 121}{6} - \frac{3600}{(6)(4)}$$

$$= \frac{1030}{6} - \frac{3600}{24}$$

$$= 171.67 - 150$$

$$= 21.67$$

Sums of Squares Within Subjects:

$$SS_{within} = \text{Total squared sums} - \frac{\text{Total subject squared sums}}{\text{treatments}}$$

$$= 180 - \frac{600}{4}$$

$$= 180 - 150$$

$$= 30$$

Computation of the Chi Square

$$\chi^2 = \frac{(\text{subjects})(\text{treatments} - 1)(SS_{treatments})}{SS_{within}}$$

$$= \frac{(6)(3)(21.67)}{30}$$

$$= \frac{390.06}{30}$$

$$= 13.00$$

Table 10.7. Data for Friedman's test. Rank order of stuttering for four verbal conditions.

Subjects	Reading Familiar Material		Singing Familiar Material		Reading Unfamiliar Material		Singing Unfamiliar Material		Total	Total^2
	Rank	R^2	Rank	R^2	Rank	R^2	Rank	R^2		
1	3	9	1	1	4	16	2	4	10	100
2	3	9	2	4	4	16	1	1	10	100
3	2	4	1	1	4	16	3	9	10	100
4	4	16	1	1	3	9	2	4	10	100
5	4	16	2	4	3	9	1	1	10	100
6	3	9	1	1	4	16	2	4	10	100
										↓
Totals $\sum R$	19		8		22		11		60	600
$\sum R^2$		63		12		82		23	180	
$(\sum R)^2$	361		64		484		121		360	

Grand Total = 60
Subjects = 6
Treatments = 4
Total Squared Sums = 180
Total Subject Squared Sums = 600

Degrees of Freedom = treatments − 1

$$= 4 - 1$$
$$= 3$$

χ^2 value for $df = 3$, $p. < .01 = 11.3$

The present result of 13.0 exceeds the 11.3 necessary for significance, as listed in the table of Chi Square values (see Appendix I). Therefore, the difference in rankings of stuttering during the four conditions is significant. Observation of the ranks indicates that least stuttering appeared during the singing of familiar lyrics, while the most stuttering appeared during the reading of unfamiliar lyrics. As a follow-up test (post hoc) for the difference between individual conditions, Healey *et al.* used the Wilcoxon Matched Pairs Test, which is described in the previous section.

CHAPTER 11 Multiple Comparison Tests with Two or More Factors

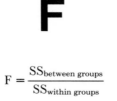

$$F = \frac{SS_{\text{between groups}}}{SS_{\text{within groups}}}$$

TWO FACTOR ANALYSIS OF VARIANCE WITH REPEATED MEASURES ON ONE FACTOR

(Treatments-by-Groups)

A test for differences among normally distributed variables.

Two or more groups of subjects are given several tests (treatments).

Each subject takes all tests.

The F results answer these questions:

1. Is there a difference between groups?
2. Is there a difference between treatments?
3. Is there an interaction between groups and treatments?

Data Arrangement:

Subjects	Treatment 1	Treatment 2	Treatment 3

Group 1 1
          2
          3
          4			

Group 2 1
          2
          3
          4			

Figure 11.1. Data arrangement for the treatment-by-groups design.

Quite often the *types* of subjects used in the experiment are a critical part of the research question. In the speech, language, and hearing field, researchers are typically concerned about subcategories such as different kinds of aphasics, different age levels of language development, males compared to females, or types of hearing loss. Since each group of subjects is to be tested by several measures, the two factor design is needed.

This procedure is, in a sense, like stacking two treatments-by-subjects tests on top of each other. The advantage of making one big analysis instead of two smaller ones is to test the *interactions*. This is a cumbersome term to explain, but it means that although one group may perform generally better than the other, the difference is not consistent—some tests show a much bigger difference than others. When this inconsistency occurs the analysis shows a *significant interaction*. For instance, older children will score higher on a language test than will young children, but the main difference may be for verbs rather than for nouns. A significant F for the interaction indicates that this uneven difference is big enough to influence the overall test results.

Computational Example

For our example of this statistic, a study by Cecconi *et al.* (1977) was designed to test the fluency of normal children during the oral reading of five different levels of difficulty in reading material. One part of the study was to compare the performance of male and female speakers at the different reading levels. For a simplified analogy of the study our fictitious data are arranged (Table 11.1) to display the performance of males and females at three levels of oral reading.

Completion of the Data Table

Before setting up the F test formulas, considerable time and confusion can be avoided by first computing all of the necessary values directly from the

Table 11.1 Computation of the treatments-by-groups analysis of variance. Disfluencies of males and females during three levels of oral reading.

		Reading Levels						Subject Totals	Subject Totals Squared
		Easy		Average		Hard			
	Subjects	X	X²	X	X²	X	X²		
Male	1	4	16	5	25	6	36	15	225
	2	5	25	6	36	7	49	18	324
	3	5	25	6	36	7	49	18	324
	4	4	16	7	49	9	81	20	400
Subtotals		18		24		29		71	
Female	1	5	25	6	36	8	64	19	361
	2	4	16	5	25	6	36	15	225
	3	4	16	5	25	6	36	15	225
	4	3	9	4	16	7	49	14	196
Subtotals		16		20		27		63	
Treatment Totals		34		44		56	=	134	2280
(Totals)²		1156		1936		3136	=	6228	
Squared Scores Totals			148		248		400	=	796

table. Special care should be taken at this step to be sure that each of the values is derived precisely from the correct data group.

Subjects per group = 4
Groups = 2
Treatments = 3
(Grand total)^2 = $(134)^2$ = 17956

$\sum$(each group total^2) = $(71)^2$ + $(63)^2$ = 9010
$\sum$(each subject total^2) = 2280
$\sum$(each treatment subtotal^2) = $(18)^2$ + $(24)^2$ + $(29)^2$ + $(16)^2$ + $(20)^2$ + $(27)^2$
    = 3126
$\sum$(each treatment total^2) = 6228
$\sum$(each score^2) = 796

Computation of the F Results

Step 1. Sums of Squares Between Groups of Subjects

$SS_{\text{between groups}}$

$$= \frac{\sum(\text{each group total}^2)}{(\text{subjects per group})(\text{treatments})}$$

$$- \frac{(\text{grand total})^2}{(\text{subjects per group})(\text{groups})(\text{treatments})}$$

$$= \frac{(71)^2 + (63)^2}{(4)(3)} - \frac{(134)^2}{(4)(2)(3)}$$

$$= \frac{5041 + 3969}{12} - \frac{17956}{24}$$

$$= 750.83 - 748.17$$

$$= 2.66$$

Step 2. Sums of Squares Within Groups of Subjects

$SS_{\text{within groups}}$

$$= \frac{\sum(\text{each subject total}^2)}{\text{treatments}} - \frac{\sum(\text{each group total}^2)}{(\text{subjects per group})(\text{treatments})}$$

$$= \frac{2280}{3} - \frac{17956}{(4)(3)}$$

$$= 760.0 - 750.83$$

$$= 9.17$$

Step 3. Sums of Squares Between Treatments

$$SS_{\text{between treatments}} = \frac{\sum(\text{each treatment total}^2)}{(\text{subjects per group})(\text{groups})}$$

$$- \frac{(\text{grand total})^2}{(\text{subjects per group})(\text{groups})(\text{treatment})}$$

$$= \frac{(34)^2 + (44)^2 + (56)^2}{(4)(2)} - \frac{(134)^2}{(4)(2)(3)}$$

$$= 778.50 - 748.17$$

$$= 30.33$$

Step 4. Sums of Squares for Groups-by-Treatments Interaction

$SS_{\text{groups} \times \text{treatments}}$

$$= \frac{\Sigma(\text{each treatment subtotal}^2)}{\text{subjects per group}} - \frac{\Sigma(\text{each group total}^2)}{(\text{subjects per group})(\text{treatments})}$$

$$- \frac{\Sigma(\text{each treatment total}^2)}{(\text{subjects per group})(\text{groups})}$$

$$+ \frac{(\text{grand total})^2}{(\text{subjects per group})(\text{groups})(\text{treatments})}$$

$$= \frac{3126}{4} - \frac{9010}{(4)(3)} - \frac{6228}{(4)(2)} + \frac{17956}{(4)(2)(3)}$$

$$= 781.50 - 750.83 - 778.50 + 748.17$$

$$= .34$$

Step 5. Sums of Squares Within Treatments

$SS_{\text{within treatments}}$

$$= \Sigma(\text{each score}^2) - \frac{\Sigma(\text{each treatment subtotal}^2)}{\text{subjects per group}}$$

$$- \frac{\Sigma(\text{each subject total}^2)}{\text{treatments}} + \frac{\Sigma(\text{each group total}^2)}{(\text{subjects per group})(\text{treatments})}$$

$$= 796 - \frac{3126}{4} - \frac{2280}{3} + \frac{9010}{(4)(3)}$$

$$= 5.33$$

Degrees of Freedom

$SS_{\text{between groups}}$ df = groups $- 1 = 2 - 1 = 1$
$SS_{\text{within groups}}$ df = (groups)(subjects per group $- 1$) = $(2)(4 - 1) = 6$
$SS_{\text{between treatments}}$ df = treatments $- 1 = 3 - 1 = 2$
$SS_{\text{groups} \times \text{treatments}}$ df = (groups $- 1$)(treatments $- 1$) = $(2 - 1)(3 - 1) = 2$
$SS_{\text{within treatments}}$ df = (groups)(subjects per group $- 1$)(treatments $- 1$)
$\qquad\qquad = (2)(4 - 1)(3 - 1) = 12$

Mean Squares

$$\text{Mean Squares} = \frac{\text{Sums of Squares}}{\text{degrees of freedom}}$$

$$MS_{\text{between groups}} = \frac{2.66}{1} = 2.66$$

$$MS_{\text{within groups}} = \frac{9.17}{6} = 1.52$$

$$MS_{\text{between treatments}} = \frac{30.33}{2} = 15.16$$

$$MS_{\text{within treatments}} = \frac{5.33}{12} = .44$$

$$MS_{\text{groups-by-treatments}} = \frac{.34}{2} = .17$$

F Results

Difference between groups

$$F = \frac{MS_{\text{between groups}}}{MS_{\text{within groups}}} = \frac{2.66}{1.52} = 1.74$$

Difference between treatments

$$F = \frac{MS_{\text{between treatments}}}{MS_{\text{within treatments}}} = \frac{15.17}{.44} = 34.45$$

Groups-by-treatments Interaction

$$F = \frac{MS_{\text{groups-by-treatments}}}{MS_{\text{within treatments}}} = \frac{.17}{.44} = .39$$

Results of this analysis of variance are described in terms of the three F values. The F between groups, with a value of 1.74, was far short of the 5.99 needed for significance at the .05 level of confidence. It is therefore concluded that, although the males displayed slightly more nonfluencies than did the females, the difference between the groups was not significant. A significant difference, however, was found among the three levels of difficulty in the oral reading material (F = 34.45; df = 2, 12; p. < .01). Mean disfluencies computed from our data for the three reading levels were 4.25, 5.50, and 7.00, revealing that disfluency tends to increase with difficulty of material, as reported by Cecconi *et al.* Finally, the groups-by-treatments interaction was not significant (F = .39 did not exceed the 3.55 necessary for significance at .05 level, with 2 and 12 degrees of freedom), indicating that male and female disfluencies were comparable at each reading level.

In this example the point has been made, by the significant F between treatments, that disfluencies tend to increase as reading material difficulty increases, and further analysis of the data is unnecessary. However, in

Table 11.2 Summary table for the treatments-by-groups analysis of variance.

Source of Variation	SS	df	MS	F
Between Groups	2.66	1	2.66	1.74
Within Groups	9.1	6	1.52	
Between Treatments	30.33	2	15.16	34.45
Within Treatments	5.33	12	1.49	
Groups-by-Treatments	.33	2	.16	.39

situations where specific differences between individual groups or treatments are critical in drawing conclusions, post hoc analysis following a significant F would be used. These techniques are described in the section which follows the analyses of variance.

F

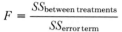

$$F = \frac{SS_{\text{between treatments}}}{SS_{\text{error term}}}$$

TWO FACTOR ANALYSIS OF VARIANCE WITH REPEATED MEASURES OF BOTH FACTORS

(Treatments-by-Treatments-by-Subjects AOV)

A test for differences among treatments, for two types of conditions.
This analysis yields three F scores, which answer the following questions:
1. Is there a difference between groups in treatment (condition) A?
2. Is there a difference between groups in treatment (condition) B?
3. Is there an interaction between treatments A and B?

Data should be arranged according to this chart:

Treatments A		I		II	
Treatments B	1	2	1	2	
Subjects					
1					
2					
3					
4					
5					
—					

Figure 11.2. Data arranged for the treatments-by-treatments-by-subjects analysis of variance.

The treatments-by-treatments-by-subjects analysis of variance is, as its name implies, an expansion of the simpler treatments-by-subjects analysis. In this design another treatment factor has been added, which also has subclasses. To illustrate this arrangement, if subjects were to be tested with three kinds of hearing aids, this would be a treatments-by-subjects design; if they were tested with the three aids under conditions of quiet and noise, another factor would be added, giving us a treaments-by-treatments-by-subjects design. Although the results of this statistic are based only on the two treatment factors (plus the interaction) it is sometimes treated as a three factor design. Particularly when the statistic is to be run in a computer program, the *Subjects* must be treated as a third factor, which the computer uses to categorize the error term. For hand calculator purposes, however, the Subjects part of the design need not be treated as a separate factor. For this reason we have considered the procedure to be simply a two factor repeated measures design, as presented by Myers (1972).

In the three F results from the test, comparisons within the two treatment factors are called the *main effects*. Paradoxically, the main effects do not always yield the most important results; in some studies the results of primary interest are found in the interactions.

Computational Example

Orchik *et al.* (1979) employed this version of the analysis of variance to compare the W-22 and NU-6 word lists for auditory discrimination in 30 adults having sensori-neural hearing loss. Three loudness levels were used in the tests. It was found that discrimination scores for the W-22 were significantly better at all loudness levels. For our simplified computation, fictitious data representing scores from 5 subjects will be used.

TREATMENTS-BY-TREATMENTS-BY-SUBJECTS ANALYSIS OF VARIANCE

Treatment A: Two Test Lists (NU-6 vs. W-22)
Treatment B: Two loudness Levels

$$Correction\ Term = \frac{(\text{Grand Total})^2}{\text{Total Number of Scores}}$$

Table 11.3. Computation of the T × T × S analysis of variance. Totals and squares for subjects.

Treatment A: Treatment B: Subjects	List 1				List 2				Grand Totals	
	Loudness 1		Loudness 2		Loudness 1		Loudness 2			
	X_1	$X_1{}^2$	X_2	$X_2{}^2$	X_1	$X_1{}^2$	X_2	$X_2{}^2$	ΣX	$(\Sigma X)^2$
1	1	1	7	49	3	9	7	49	18	324
2	3	9	5	25	5	25	9	81	22	484
3	3	9	3	9	5	25	7	49	18	324
4	3	9	5	25	5	25	7	49	20	400
5	5	25	5	25	7	49	5	25	22	484
Total	15		25		25		35		= 100	
Total of Squares		53		133		133		253	= 572	
Sum Squared	225		625		625		1225		= 2700	
										2016

Grand Total = 100
Total of All Squared Scores = 572
Total Subject Sums Squared = 2700
Total Subject Rows Squared = 2016
Total Number of Scores = 20
Total Number of Columns = 4
Total Number of Subjects = 5
Number of Scores in Each Part of Treatment A = 10
Number of Scores in Each Part of Treatment B = 10

Table 11.4. Totals of squares of treatment A: (two word lists).

Subjects	List 1		List 2		
	X_1	$(\Sigma X_1)^2$	X_2	$(\Sigma X_2)^2$	
1	8	64	10	100	Record the total scores for each
2	8	64	14	196	subject on each word list (treat-
3	6	36	12	144	ment A), and square these num-
4	8	75	12	144	bers.
5	10	100	12	144	
Total	40		60		= 100 = Grand Total
Total of Squares 60				728	= 1056 = Total Squared Scores A
Sum Squared 1600			3600		= 5200 = Total Sums Squared A

$$= \frac{(100)^2}{20}$$

$$= 500$$

Total Sums of Squares = Total of all Squared Scores − Correction Term

$$SS_{\text{total}} = 572 - 500$$

$$= 72$$

Sums of Squares for Subjects

$$= \frac{\text{Total Subject Rows Squared}}{\text{Total Number of Columns}} - \text{Correction Term}$$

$$SS_{\text{subjects}} = \frac{2016}{4} - 500$$

$$= 4$$

Sums of Squares for Treatment A $= \dfrac{\text{Total Sums Squared A}}{\text{Number of scores for each part of A}}$

$$- \text{Correction Term}$$

$$SS_{\text{A}} = \frac{5200}{10} - 500$$

$$= 20$$

Sums of Squares for Treatment B $= \dfrac{\text{Total Sums Squared B}}{\text{Number of scores for each part of B}}$

$$- \text{Correction Term}$$

$$SS_{\text{B}} = \frac{5200}{10} - 500$$

$$= 20$$

Sums of Squares for Treatment A × *Treatment B*

$$= \frac{\text{Total Subject Sums Squared}}{\text{Number of Subjects}} - \text{Correction Term} - SS_{\text{A}} - SS_{\text{B}}$$

$$SS_{\text{A}\times\text{B}} = \frac{2700}{5} - 500 - 20 - 20$$

$$= 0$$

Sums of Squares for Error A

$$SS_{\text{error A}} = \frac{\text{Total Squared Scores A}}{\text{Number of responses for each subject on each part of A}}$$

$$- \text{Correction Term} - SS_{\text{subjects}} - SS_{\text{A}}$$

$$= \frac{1056}{2} - 500 - 4 - 20$$

$$= 4$$

Sums of Squares for Error B

$$SS_{\text{error B}} = \frac{\text{Total Squared Scores B}}{\text{Number of responses for each subject on each part of A}}$$

$$- \text{Correction Term} - SS_{\text{subjects}} - SS_{\text{B}}$$

$$= \frac{1088}{2} - 500 - 4 - 20$$

$$= 20$$

Sums of Squares for Error A × B:

$$SS_{\text{error A} \times \text{B}} = SS_{\text{total}} - SS_{\text{subjects}} - SS_{\text{A}} - SS_{\text{B}} - SS_{\text{A} \times \text{B}} - SS_{\text{error A}} - SS_{\text{error B}}$$

$$= 72 - 4 - 20 - 20 - 0 - 4 - 20$$

$$= 4$$

Degrees of Freedom: df

$$df\ SS_{\text{total}} = \text{Categories of Treatment A} \times \text{Categories of Treatment B}$$
$$\times \text{Number of Subjects} - 1$$
$$= (2)(2)(5) - 1$$
$$= 19 = \text{Total number of scores, minus one.}$$

$$df\ SS_{\text{subjects}} = \text{Number of Subjects} - 1$$
$$= 5 - 1$$
$$= 4$$

$$df\ SS_{\text{A}} = \text{Categories of Treatment A} - 1$$
$$= 2 - 1$$
$$= 1$$

$$df\ SS_{\text{B}} = \text{Categories of Treatment B} - 1$$
$$= 2 - 1$$
$$= 1$$

$$df\ SS_{\text{A} \times \text{B}} = df\ SS_{\text{A}} \times df\ SS_{\text{B}}$$
$$= (1)(1)$$
$$= 1$$

$$df\ SS_{\text{error A}} = df\ SS_{\text{subjects}} \times df\ SS_{A}$$
$$= (4)(1)$$
$$= 4$$

$$df\ SS_{\text{error B}} = df\ SS_{\text{subjects}} \times df\ SS_{B}$$
$$= (4)(1)$$
$$= 4$$

$$df\ SS_{\text{error A}\times B} = df\ SS_{\text{subjects}} \times df\ SS_{A} \times df\ SS_{B}$$
$$= (4)(1)(1)$$
$$= 4$$

Conclusions:

Treatment A: $F = 20$; $df = 1, 4$; $p. < .05$
There is a significant difference between the two lists.
Treatment B: $F = 4$; $df = 1, 4$; $p. > .05$
There is no significant difference between loudness levels.
Interaction A × B: $F = 0$; $df = 1,4$; $p. > .05$
There is no significant interaction between treatments.

Results of the F tests indicate a significant difference in treatment A, which contains the two discrimination word lists in our example. Inspection of the

Table 11.5. Totals of squares of treatment B: (two loudness levels).

Subjects	Loudness 1 X_1	$(\Sigma X_1)^2$	Loudness 2 X_2	$(\Sigma X_2)^2$	
1	4	16	14	196	Record the total scores for each
2	8	64	14	196	subject on each loudness level
3	8	64	10	100	(treatment B), and square these
4	8	64	12	144	numbers.
5	12	144	10	100	
Total	40		60		= 100 = Grand Total
Total of Squares	352		736		= 1088 = Total Squared Scores B
Sum Squared	1600		3600		= 5200 = Total Sums Squared B

Table 11.6. Summary Table (the source table) for the T × T × S analysis of variance.

	Sums of Squares		df	Mean Squares $\dfrac{SS}{df}$	F ratio	F
SS_A	=	20	1	20	$\dfrac{20}{1}$	20
$SS_{\text{error A}}$	=	4	4	1		
SS_B	=	20	1	20	$\dfrac{20}{5}$	4
$SS_{\text{error B}}$	=	20	4	5		
$SS_{A\times B}$	=	0	1	0	$\dfrac{0}{1}$	0
$SS_{\text{error A}\times B}$	=	4	4	1		

discrimination scores for the two lists reveals better scores for List 2, which represents the W-22 sample. Since there were only two lists being tested in this example, and the other F results were not significant, further analysis is unnecessary. However, if the investigation had included four or five types of test lists, a *post hoc* analysis following the significant F would have been helpful to determine which of the lists differed from the rest.

CHAPTER 12 Transformations and Post Hoc Analysis

TRANSFORMATIONS

When groups of data are somehow unsuited to statistical analysis, the numbers can be altered (transformed) in various ways in order to improve their applicability. For example, scores which have the value of zero do not work well in statistical analysis because they can not be multiplied. It is therefore advisable to add a .5 or a 1.0 to each score in order to eliminate the zeros from the computation. As long as the same value is added to all of the scores the validity of the analysis will remain unchanged. Similarly, in order to reduce the size of large numbers to allow for simpler computation, a certain value—such as 100—could be subtracted from each score. Adding or subtracting a fixed value from each score is called an *additive transformation*.

From a more theoretical standpoint, transformations are sometimes employed prior to the computation of the analysis of variance to produce a better match of variances among the groups of data (homogeneity of variance) or to reduce skewness or bimodality of the data for a more normally distributed pattern. In some instances, this treatment of data tends to make the AOV more sensitive, therefore reducing the chance of a Type II error. In actual practice, however, the benefit from normative transformations on a routine basis is rather dubious because of the robust nature of the analysis of variance. The AOV, in other words, will yield about the same result in spite of minor deviations from normality or from homogeneity of variance. In more extreme examples, however, where the data are clearly not normally distributed, the results might better be obtained through nonparametric methods. In spite of the relatively weak pragmatic basis for the general implementation of transformations (Winer, 1971), they are needed occasionally for the fine tuning of some types of data.

Arcsin Transformations

Aside from the commonplace additive transformations mentioned previously, the arcsin (also spelled arcsine, arc-sin, or arc sine) is the only transformation which may be found regularly in the speech, language, and hearing literature. It is used rather routinely in studies where an analysis of variance is to be based upon percentage scores. As a rule, percentage scores tend to cluster at the high end of the range, rather than around the 50% area for a more standardized normal distribution. The effect of the arcsin transformation is to shift all scores downward, thereby centering the newly formed distribution around the middle percentages, as shown in the graph below.

137

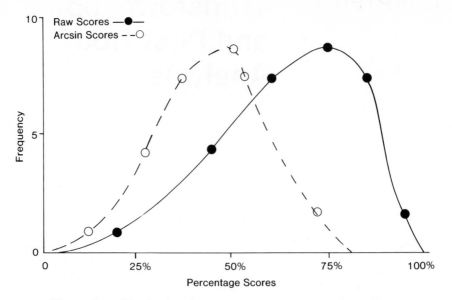

Figure 12.1. Distributions for raw scores and arcsin transformations.

Specifically, if most of the percentage scores are found to cluster around 80% (which is often the case), the arcsin transformation will shift the numbers to peak at about 50%, which would be at the center of the new distribution range (Figure 12.1).

A more versatile version of the arcsin transformation is suggested by Winer (1971), which has the effect of shifting both high and low percentage scores toward the middle of the range. The farther the scores are from the 50% midpoint of the range, the more they are moved toward the middle of the new distribution. The advantage of this transformation is that no matter what shape the percentage distribution happens to have, it will automatically be set up in relation to a theoretical population which has a mean at the 50% marker. Winer's formula incorporates both the arcsin, which shifts high percentages downward, and the square root, which shifts low percentages upward:

$$\text{Transformation} = 2 \arcsin \sqrt{X\%}$$

Tables are available for this transformation, but the formula is also well suited for the programmable calculator.

The effect of this transformation is illustrated in Figure 12.2. It should be noted that the percentage scores in the graph are skewed to the left, typical of percentage data. *Skewed* originally came from a term meaning "to swerve out of line" or "to escape." In statistics, the direction of the skew refers to the tail of the curve, so that our percentage data would be described as "skewed to the left" or "negatively skewed." It can be seen that the transformed data curve has been altered so as to peak closer to the middle of the range and that both the left and right ends of the curve are pulled toward the middle, producing a more uniform and evenly centered distribution.

In comparing the two transformation graphs, it may be seen that the simple arcsin transformation will shift all scores to the left, i.e., toward the lower percentage values. This treatment will serve very well in the rather typical situation in which the percentage scores are clustered around the upper quartile. This type of data is often found in classroom examinations, in which most of the class is apt to achieve test scores of about 75% correct answers. The rather drastic shift of the curve toward the lower percentages is employed in this situation in order to produce a more normal distribution and to eliminate the long tail skewed to the left of the original data. In the second chart, a more gentle shift of the data is seen, which tends to bring all of the data somewhat closer toward the middle and reduces the skewness of the curve by shifting the left side up closer to the mean. Since both the high and low extremes are minimized by this treatment, it can be viewed as a general purpose type of transformation which will make all types of distributions fall into a more equitable pattern for comparative analysis.

In published articles we may assume that many examples of transformed data are not mentioned in the procedural part of the report. The technique of adding a .5 or a 1 to all scores in order to eliminate zeros is perhaps too obvious a detail to be included in the report. Similarly, other types of transformations might also be treated as minor steps in the analysis, or even as an incidental part of the computer progam. Arcsin transformations, however, tend to have a special role in the treatment of percentage data, and are therefore viewed as standard recommended procedure by many journal editors for this type of analysis.

In a study to compare responses to time-compressed verbal material by reading-impaired and normal-reading children, Freeman and Beasley (1978) tabulated the percentage of correct responses for each child. "To avoid difficulties associated with skewness of percentage-correct scores, statistical analyses were accomplished using arc sine transformations of individual scores" (*ibid*, p. 499). The analysis of variance which followed the transformation treatment indicated that reading-impaired children have more difficulty in processing complex linguistic stimuli.

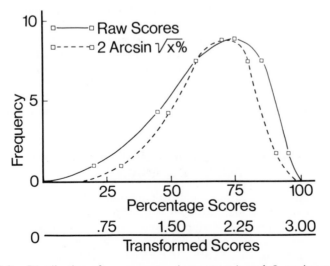

Figure 12.2. Distributions for raw scores (percentages) and 2 arcsin-square root transformations.

Two additional studies which illustrate the use of arcsin transformations deal with the word-recognition abilities of aphasics. One study (Mills *et al.*, 1979) recorded the percentage of errors made by aphasics and normals to material having varying degrees of uncertainty. The other (Zurif *et al.*, 1979) recorded the percentage of correct word identifications from two types of aphasics and normals. In both examples, arcsin transformations were considered necessary for better distribution of the percentage data prior to computation of the analysis of variance.

Square Root Transformations

In a sense, the square root transformation is the mirror image of the arcsin transformation, in that it shifts low scores upward in the same manner that the arcsin transformation shifts high scores downward. It follows then that square root treatment of the data will normalize distributions which are composed primarily of small numbers. With numbers which are mostly below 10, especially if some zeros are included, the formula:

$$\text{Transformation} = \sqrt{X + .5}$$

is recommended. Examples of this transformation are not readily found in the communication disorders literature, but it would be of obvious benefit in normalizing data based on the number of errors from relatively simple testing methods. With this type of data, most subjects would make very few errors and some would probably make no errors at all. The square root transformation to all data groups prior to the analysis of variance would make the analysis slightly more sensitive in detecting significant differences.

Logarithmic Transformations

The most familiar example of the logarithmic transformation is the audiogram, in which the higher frequencies are compressed, and the low frequencies are more widely spaced. The effect of the transformation is to denote more importance to differences in low frequencies, and to indicate that a very large frequency shift is needed before it is noticed in the high frequencies. Other types of chart paper are based upon the logarithmic transformation, in which a difference of five or ten points means a lot among small scores, but makes very little difference among very high scores. For statistical analysis, this transformation finds some usage in equating groups of data in which the variance increases as the mean increases, or in straightening some curvilinear regression lines for the purpose of multiple correlation. Logarithmic values for this transformation are available on many inexpensive models of pocket calculators.

COMPARISONS FOLLOWING ANALYSIS OF VARIANCE: POST HOC ANALYSIS

Since the analysis of variance tells us only that at least one among all the possible comparisons is significant, it is sometimes important to determine which differences specifically were responsible for the significant result. To accomplish this purpose, we find that several techniques appear regularly in the research literature. These are often referred to as *multiple comparison tests*, indicating that all comparisons can be achieved through a single procedure. The tests, using some of the results computed during the analysis of variance, establish a criterion score which is used as a "yardstick" in determining which differences are significant and which are not. Any differences exceeding the *critical value* are considered to be significant. In general, multiple comparison tests are fairly easy to compute and efficient, since they employ information "left over" from the AOV.

Three of the most common multiple comparison tests are the Newman-Keuls, the Scheffé, and the Tukey test. Even though these tests do approximately the same thing, they are not equally sensitive and may serve slightly different needs. The most conservative is the Scheffé. This test should be used when only the fewest number of significant comparisons are needed in the results. Some studies, however, are intended to show the maximum number of significant comparisons. In this case, the Newman-Keuls should be used instead of the Scheffé.

For a general purpose test, considered to be the best compromise between one which might be too conservative and one which might be too liberal, the Tukey test is recommended. This test is not found frequently in the earlier literature, but more recent research articles display increasing use of the Tukey for post hoc analysis.

t-Tests for Post Hoc Analysis

In addition to the multiple comparison tests, the *t*-test is also used to find which groups are significantly different following a significant *F* result. Generally speaking the multiple comparison tests are preferable to the *t*-test for post hoc analysis, but on some occasions the *t*-test is useful, even though it has two disadvantages:

1. Multiple *t*-tests run a greater risk of error than do multiple comparison tests. While the statistical probability of error increases with each additional *t*-test run on the same *F* test data, the multiple comparison tests can be used on any number of pairs without changing the probability level.

2. Multiple *t*-tests are much more tedious to perform than are the multiple comparisons.

When relatively few *t*-tests need to be run, however, the computational inconvenience becomes negligible, particularly if they can be set up on a programmable calculator. Some post hoc analyses do not require that all comparisons must be made, since the final result of the study is concerned only with certain areas of special interest. In this situation, a few *t*-tests can be made rather easily, with the rest of the possible comparisons being ignored. However, the *t*-test should not be over-used with the same data groups. It should be limited to relatively few tests—preferably less than ten—and should be used with a conservative probability for error, such as .01 or .001.

Post Hoc Analysis of Interactions

The analysis of specific comparisons which account for a significant *F* in interactions is not well discussed in statistical texts, and is sometimes the source of confusion. The best insight into interactive effects in the *F* test may be gained by plotting the means on chart paper. In many cases, this type of analysis is sufficient, together with the visual inspection of which means display the greatest difference. This part of the result is usually described along with the *F* ratios in the results section of the report and is not necessarily accompanied by additional computation.

However, in some reports, particularly where the interactive effects are the focal point of the study, the post hoc analysis is extended to include this part of the F results. In these comparisons, all means in the interaction might be significantly different, but the problem is to find which means differ more than the others. One approach is to use a series of t-tests which are set at a high probability level, in order to screen out only those comparisons which have the greatest differences. A more efficient way is to treat all possible comparisons with a single multivariate analysis, available as a computer program.

Nonparametric Tests

The nonparametric versions of the analyses of variance are the Kruskal-Wallis H as the one factor AOV for independent measures, and the Friedman Test as the treatments-by-subjects AOV for related measures. Post hoc analysis for these tests are also nonparametric techniques. Tests for specific differences among the groups of the Kruskal-Wallis H may be derived through use of the Mann-Whitney U. Similarly, specific differences in the Friedman Test are found by use of the Wilcoxon Matched Pairs T test.

TUKEY TEST

Critical Value $= (q)$(Standard Error)

As indicated in the formula shown above, the Tukey Test provides a critical value or "yardstick" for comparing any of the two means involved in the overall analysis of variance. Both the q and the standard error are easily obtained, and the critical value is easily computed. The q value is obtained from a table of the *Studentized Range Statistic*, and is determined by the total number of means in the set, and by the degrees of freedom in the error term of the AOV. In our present example, the sums of squares within groups (SS_{within}) is the error term.

Using the data from the one way analysis of variance described earlier, the following F summary will be used for the Tukey Test (Table 12.1):
The analysis is based upon the comprehension scores of three age groups. The means for the three groups are:

Age 4 = 3.40   Age 6 = 7.20   Age 8 = 7.80

There are five children in each group.

Computation of the Tukey Test

q Value

For determining the q value there are three means (age groups) in the set, and the sums of squares within groups has 12 degrees of freedom. The number of means is considered to be the range, using the symbol r for the table. From the table of the Studentized Range, the q value for $r = 3$ and df = 12 is 3.77 at the .05 level.

Table 12.1. Summary table for the one-way analysis of variance.

Source of Variation	df	Sum of Squares	Mean Squares	F
$SS_{between}$	2	56.93	28.47	14.98
SS_{within}	12	22.80	1.90	

Standard Error

The second value is determined by the error term and by the number of scores per group. In our error term is the mean squares within groups, which is 1.90, and there are five scores per group. With these numbers the standard error is computed by:

$$\text{Standard Error} = \sqrt{\frac{\text{MS}_{\text{within}} \text{ error term}}{\text{scores per group}}}$$

$$= \sqrt{\frac{1.9}{5}}$$

$$= .62$$

The Tukey test is now computed as:

$$\textit{Critical Difference} = (q)(\text{standard error})$$

$$= (3.77)(.62)$$

$$= 2.34$$

If the difference between any of the mean is greater than the critical value of 2.32, the difference is significant at the .05 level of confidence.

Age 4 vs. age 6 = 7.20 − 3.40 = 3.80 (significant)

Age 4 vs. age 8 = 7.80 − 3.40 = 4.40 (significant)

Age 6 vs. age 8 = 7.80 − 7.20 = .60 (not significant)

The significance level for the Tukey test is usually set at the .05 level. As mentioned earlier, among the various multiple comparison tests the Tukey test seems to be the best compromise, in that it tends to yield perhaps the most realistic number of mean differences. On the basis of the Tukey test, it is determined that there is a significant difference between the mean scores for ages 4–6, and between ages 4–8. The difference between ages 6–8 is not significant.

THE SCHEFFÉ TEST

Critical Difference = (Standard Error)(F Factor)

The Scheffé approach to post hoc comparisons following analysis of variance is one of the earliest of the widely used treatments. Although the Scheffé still appears regularly in the literature, it is now used selectively, rather than as the common standard method. Its primary value is where a very conservative result is needed, showing only the most prominent significant comparisons within the analysis of variance groups. In addition to being more conservative than either the Tukey or the Newman-Keuls tests, it utilizes a somewhat different formula, based upon the F table rather than the Studentized Range q table used by the other multiple comparison methods. A unique feature of the Scheffé is that it has the capability of lumping several groups together in the comparisons, as well as performing the usual test for differences between individual means.

Computational Example

A one-way simple analysis of variance comparing the difference among the three means yielded a significant F test result at the .01 probability level (Table 12.3).

Since the F test result is significant, we know that there is a significant difference between at least two of the delayed feedback conditions. Inspection of the data (Table 12.2) shows that the biggest difference is between the .5 delay (Group A) and the .25 delay condition (Group C) and we can therefore assume that this difference is significant. However, we do not know if there are other significant differences among the three conditions. The Scheffé Test will be computed to check for a difference between Group A and Group B. Further comparison will be made between Group A and Groups B and C combined.

Four numerical values are needed in order to compute the Scheffé. These are described by different names and different symbols, and there is unfortunately no consistancy from one reference book to the next. The first of these values is the *Group Weight Factor*, which serves to modify the statistic according to the number of subjects in the groups to be compared.

Group Weight Factor:

$$\frac{1}{\text{Number of scores in the mean for the first group}} + \frac{1}{\text{Number of scores in the mean for the second group}}$$

In this case there are 6 subjects in each group to be compared.

$$\frac{1}{6} + \frac{1}{6} = \frac{1}{3}$$

The second value is an estimate of the standard deviation of the two comparison groups, or in other words, the *standard error*.

Table 12.2. Raw data for the Scheffé test. Nonfluency during oral readings for three delay settings of DAF.

Subjects	A .5 sec	B .33 sec	C .25 sec
1	4	0	1
2	5	2	0
3	3	1	0
4	3	2	1
5	4	2	2
6	2	2	2
Totals	21	9	6
Means	3.5	1.5	1.0

Table 12.3. Summary table for the one-way analysis of variance.

Source	Sum of Squares	Degrees of Freedom	Mean Squares	F
Between Conditions	21	2	10.5	12.1
Within Conditions	13	15	0.867	
Total	34	17		

Standard Error:

$$= \sqrt{\text{(Group Weight Factor) (Mean Squares Error Term,} \atop \text{from the AOV results)}}$$

$$= \sqrt{(1/3)(.867)}$$

$$= \sqrt{\frac{.867}{3}}$$

$$= \sqrt{.2890} = .5376$$

F Factor:

$$= \sqrt{\left(\begin{matrix}\text{Number of groups in} \\ \text{the AOV, minus 1}\end{matrix}\right)\left(\begin{matrix}\text{Selected} \\ F\text{ Value}\end{matrix}\right)}$$

$$= \sqrt{(3 - 1)(3.68)}$$

$$= \sqrt{7.36}$$

$$= 2.71$$

In this example, the F value was selected at the .05 confidence level, with 2 and 15 degrees of freedom. F value is selected from the F table for groups-1 as the df numerator, with df error term as the denominator.

Critical Value:

$$= \text{(Standard Error)}(F\text{ Factor)}$$

$$= (5.376)(2.71)$$

$$= 1.46$$

If the obtained difference between two means in the AOV is greater than the critical value of 1.46 it is significant at the .05 confidence level.

Group A vs. B: difference between means is 2.0; significant at .01

Group A vs. C: difference between means is 2.5; significant at .01

Group B vs. C: difference between means is   .5; not significant

This completes the comparison between all possible individual group means in the AOV. In some cases, however, it may be important to combine the means of one or more of the groups in order to look for differences in broader categories. Using the present example, Group A will be compared with the combined condition of the B and C groups.

$$\text{A vs. B and C groups} = \frac{\text{Mean for A group}}{\text{Number of means shown above}}$$

$$- \frac{\text{Means for B + C}}{\text{Number of means shown above}}$$

$$= \frac{3.5}{1} - \frac{15. + 1.0}{2}$$

$$= 3.5 - 1.25$$

$$= 2.25 = \text{difference to be tested}$$

Group Weight Factor $= \dfrac{1}{n} + \dfrac{1}{n}$

$$1/6 + 1/12 = 3/12 = 1/4 = .25$$

Standard Error $= \sqrt{(\text{Group Weight Factor})(\text{error term})}$

$$\sqrt{(.25)(.867)} = \sqrt{.217} = .465$$

F Factor $= \sqrt{(\text{Groups-1})(F\ .05)}$

$$\sqrt{(3 - 1)(3.68)} = 2.713$$

Critical Difference $=$ (Standard Error)(F Factor)

$$(.465)(2.713) = 1.26$$

Result: The 2.25 difference in the A vs. B + C comparison is greater than the critical difference value of 1.26, and it is therefore significant at the .05 confidence level. The same computational procedure using the .01 level may also be used, and the choice between .01 and .05 is a matter of how conservative the researcher feels the results should be. The .05 will usually yield more significant differences than will the .01.

NEWMAN-KEULS TEST FOR MULTIPLE COMPARISONS

Critical Difference $= (q)$ (Standard Error)

At the present time, the Newman-Keuls is the most frequently used multiple comparison test, following a significant analysis of variance F result. The Tukey Test, however, is often recommended as the best choice for general use, and the Newman-Keuls might therefore be replaced eventually by the Tukey as the most common post hoc method. Like the Tukey Test, the Newman-Keuls also uses the q value to derive the Critical Difference. However, the Newman-Keuls is based upon the number of means which separate each comparison, while the Tukey uses the total number of means in the factor being compared. The Newman-Keuls will yield more significant differences than will the Tukey or Scheffé, assuming that all tests are used with a probability level of .05.

Computational Example

In a study to determine the effects of masking and delayed auditory feedback upon stuttering, Stephen and Haggard (1980) used the Newman-Keuls test to discover which types of masking and DAF showed significant differences, as indicated by the significant F result. It was found that masking and DAF produced an increase in reading rate, accompanied by a decrease in stuttering. Intermittent masking produced more fluency than did continuous masking. For our simplified example, we shall present fictitious scores of stuttering blocks from 11 stutterers under three conditions of the masking factor.

Data

Mean Number of Blocks Under Three Conditions For a Group of 11 Stutterers

	A No Masking	B Continuous Masking	C Intermittent Masking
Means	12	7	4
Rank Order	1	2	3

Analysis of Variance Summary

	df	Mean Squares	F
Between Treatments	2	33.50	12.36
Residual Error Term	20	2.71	

Standard Error

In computing the Standard Error, the Mean Squares error term value from the analysis of variance summary is used.

$$\text{Standard Error} = \sqrt{\frac{\text{Mean Squares}_{\text{error term}}}{\text{subjects per group}}}$$

$$= \sqrt{\frac{2.71}{11}}$$

$$= .50$$

q Value

The q value is taken from the Table of the Studentized Range, using $r =$ range of ranks being compared, and $df =$ degrees of freedom of the error term in the AOV summary. In this example of $df = 20$, $p. = .01$.

$$\text{For } r = 2, q = 4.02$$

$$\text{For } r = 3, q = 4.64$$

Critical Difference

The q value and the standard error for each comparison have already been calculated in the preceding steps. The Standard Error remains the same for all Critical Difference computations, but the q value changes with the range across which each comparison is to be made.

Critical Difference Across 2 Ranks:

$$= (q) \text{ (Standard Error)}$$

$$= 4.02)(.50)$$

$$= 2.01$$

Critical Difference Across 3 Ranks:

$$= (4.64)(.50)$$

$$= 2.32$$

Applying the Newman-Keuls Comparisons

The difference between means and the range of means across each comparison should first be established. Note that the range determines which Critical Difference should be used. If the difference between two means exceeds the Critical Difference, the group difference is significant.

Comparison	Range	Group Difference	Critical Difference
Group A—Group B	2	$12 - 7 = 5$ (Sig,.05)	2.01
Group A—Group C	3	$12 - 4 = 8$ (Sig,.05)	2.32
Group B—Group C	2	$7 - 4 = 3$ (Sig,.05)	2.01

On the basis of the Newman-Keuls post hoc analysis it was found that stutterers have significantly fewer blocks ($p. < .01$) in either of the masking conditions than were exhibited in the unmasked condition. Further, the intermittent masking condition resulted in significantly fewer blocks than were found during continuous masking, as reported by Stephen and Haggard (1980).

CHAPTER 13　**Correlations**

r

PEARSON PRODUCT-MOMENT CORRELATION

A correlation statistic is to determine the relationship of one variable to another. In other words, it is an indication of how well a score from one set of measures will predict the equivalent score on another set of measures. Its result is in the form of a coefficient value which may vary from 1.00, a perfect positive correlation, to a −1.00, which is a perfect negative correlation. A result of .00 indicates a complete lack of relationship between the two variables.

The assumptions for use of the Pearson r are that the two variables are linearly related and that both have normal distribution of data. From these two rather broad assumptions a number of precautionary statements may be made.

The r result can be misleading when:
1. the relationship is not linear
2. too few measures are used
3. the samples are too selective to represent the full population

The best way to determine linear relationship is to select a small random sample of pairs of data and plot a scattergram. Visual inspection of the scattergram will not only reveal whether the data points tend to form a straight line, but will also provide a rough estimate of the resulting r value. The more the dots form a slender line, the closer the r will approach the value of 1.00. The more the dots tend to form a round circle, the closer the r will be to .00. Some relationships are not linear; height and age for example does not conform to a straight line if the elderly population is included. When the relationship is not linear the resulting r coefficient becomes smaller.

Since the rationale of the Pearson r implies that highly correlated scores will be the same distance from the means of their respective data sets, the result will be distorted if the two groups do not have the same kind of distribution.

Maximum precision of the r is obtained where both groups have the same range and standard deviation. From a practical standpoint, however, normal distribution can be assumed for most types of random samples. Sample size, however, is related to the assurance of normal distribution, and the r statistic is therefore best suited for large samples; i.e., 60 or more pairs of scores. As the number of pairs becomes less than 30, particular attention should be paid to the normalcy of the distribution. With fewer than 15 pairs of scores, or any other suggestion that the distribution may not be normal, the Spearman Rho (which is a very good nonparametric alternative) should be considered.

Finally, the accuracy of the raw score measurements should be understood as another potential source of inaccuracy for the r result. Since the r is, in a sense, a measure of random variability, it is also effected by the relative precision of the measuring method. Assuming that the two variables are actually related, an imprecise measuring technique will result in a lower r coefficient because of the unnecessary variability introduced into raw score values. Therefore, in instances where the r seems to be unrealistically low, a more exact measure of the data may yield a more satisfactory result.

Computational Example

Hollien (1962) employed the Pearson r to determine the inverse relationship between vocal cord thickness and fundamental frequency in six speakers. He

Table 13.1. Data for the Pearson r.

Frequency in Hz*		Thickness in mm.		
X	X^2	Y	Y^2	XY
02	4	9.9	98.0	19.80
05	25	9.7	94.1	48.50
10	100	8.8	77.4	88.0
15	225	9.6	92.2	144.0
20	400	8.8	77.4	176.0
21	441	9.2	84.6	193.2
23	529	8.6	74.0	197.8
24	576	8.1	65.6	194.4
25	625	7.9	62.4	197.5
26	676	8.6	74.0	223.6
27	729	8.6	74.0	232.2
30	900	7.8	60.8	234.0
35	1225	7.7	59.3	269.5
40	1600	7.6	57.8	304.0
45	2025	7.0	49.0	315.0
348	10080	127.9	1100.6	2837.5
ΣX	ΣX^2	ΣY	ΣY^2	ΣXY

* In order to reduce the numerical magnitude of these measures for easier computation, 100 Hz has been subtracted from all fundamental frequencies. This transformation has no effect on the r result.

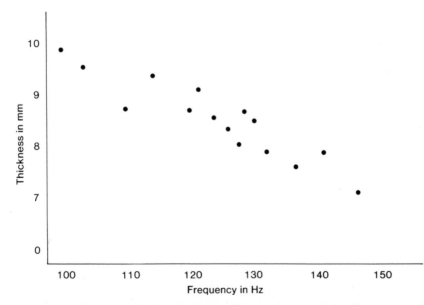

Figure 13.1. Hypothetical data depicting the negative correlation between vocal frequency and vocal cord thickness.

observed that the thickness of the vocal cords increased as the fundamental of the speakers was lowered, yielding a correlation of −.92. Each speaker was required to phonate at six prescribed pitch levels, producing a total of 36 pairs of measures from the whole group. Corresponding vocal cord thickness was measured from frontal X-ray pictures taken during phonation.

In order to simplify the computational example, 15 pairs of hypothetical measures will be used (Table 13.1).

The scattergram, which is an optional step in the r calculation, is presented to illustrate its usefulness in estimating the final outcome of the r result (Figure 13.1). In addition, as mentioned earlier, the scattergram is a check of the linear relationship between the two variables. Should the scattergram display a curve instead of a fairly straight line the r result will be at a lower value. An optional statistic which is suitable for curvilinear relationships is the *correlation ratio*.

Employing one of the most commonly used procedures, we compute the Pearson r by what is commonly termed the *machine formula*.

$$r = \frac{(N)(\Sigma XY) - (\Sigma X)(\Sigma Y)}{\sqrt{[(N)(\Sigma X^2) - (\Sigma X)^2][(N)(\Sigma Y^2) - (\Sigma Y^2)^2]}}$$

$$= \frac{(15)(2837.5) - (348)(127.9)}{\sqrt{[(15)(10080) - (348)^2][(15)(1100.6) - (127.9)^2]}}$$

$$= \frac{42562.5 - 44509.2}{\sqrt{(151200 - 121104)(16509 - 16358.4)}}$$

$$= \frac{-1946.7}{\sqrt{4532156.6}}$$

$$= -.91$$

In the formula, it does not matter whether the relationship between the two variables is positive or negative. The −.92 indicates that measures of pitch and vocal cord thickness have a highly negative correlation, as reported by Hollien.

rho

SPEARMAN RHO

$$\text{rho} = \frac{(\text{Differences in Rank})^2}{N^2}$$

The rank order correlation method is used when the data are already in the form of ranks or when the data are not normally distributed. In this latter situation the lack of normal distribution will make the data inappropriate for the Pearson r, and the raw scores may then be transformed into ranks for use with the rho statistic. The rho makes no assumption about the type of data distribution, and is an excellent alternative to the Pearson r. If the data are normally distributed, the rho and r will yield about the same correlation coefficient, with the r being perhaps slightly higher. The r however is adversely effected by unevevn variations in the data, particularly with smaller samples, and the rho becomes more accurate than the r under these conditions.

If the correlation is very high the rho may be used with as few as 6 pairs of scores. As a general rule, however, at least 10 pairs should be used in order to assure adequate significance of the result.

Computational Example

Our computational example is based upon a study by Sklar (1963) in which the relative post-mortem deterioration of cerebral cortexes were arranged in rank order to determine their relationship to test scores achieved

Table 13.2. Data for the Spearman Rho.

Observation	Cortex Rank$_1$	Weschler Test Rank$_2$	Difference $R_1 - R_2$	Difference^2
1	1	2.5	−1.5	2.25
2	2	2.5	− .5	.25
3	3	1	2	4.0
4	4	4	0	0
5	5	5	0	0
6	6	6	0	0
7	7	7	0	0
8	8	8	0	0
9	9	10	−1	1
10	10	9	1	1

$N = 10$ $\Sigma D^2 = 8.50$

$$\text{Rho} = 1 - \frac{6\Sigma D^2}{N(N^2 - 1)}$$

$$= 1 - \frac{(6)\,(8.50)}{10\,(100 - 1)}$$

$$= 1 - \frac{51}{990}$$

$$= .95$$

during the life of those individuals. The Weschler scores from the group were also transformed into rank order data to permit computation of the rho. Sklar reported a correlation of .97 for the twelve subjects represented in his study. Our hypothetical data will be based upon ten subjects (Table 13.2).

Although tables are available for determining the significance of any rho correlation coefficient, it is usually not necessary to check the probability when the correlation is high. When there are 10 or more pairs of scores and the correlation is .75 or higher, the result is significant at better than the .01 level of confidence. The rho of .95 in the present example indicates a high correlation between Weschler scores and brain condition. It implies that if either type of information is known about an individual, the other information can be predicted.

χ^2

THE 2 × 2 CHI SQUARE FOR THE RELATIONSHIP BETWEEN TWO BINOMIAL FACTORS

One of the most common forms of the chi square in speech and hearing research is called the *two-by-two* or the *fourfold chi square*. This design is used to test for the interaction between two binomial measures. The table in which this type of problem is arranged is called a *contingency table*. The degrees of freedom in the 2 × 2 arrangement are always df = 1.

As a general rule, the chi square statistic is not well suited for computation with very small groups. It is preferable to use the 2 × 2 table with an expected frequency of 10 observations per cell, or in other words at least 40 observations for the total computation. If the count falls much below 40, a correction factor known as *Yate's correction* may be used. Basically this procedure is to subtract .5 from each observation larger than expected, and to add .5 to each observation smaller than expected. If the total observations are fewer than 20, the 2 × 2 chi square should probably not be used, even with the correction factor, because the end result can now be influenced too much by a single observation.

Computational Example

Sheehan and Martyn (1970) wished to determine whether or not recovery from stuttering was associated with having received public school speech therapy. They divided a group of 112 stutterers into two types: (1) those who had received speech therapy, and (2) those who had not. All stutterers where then classed according to (1) those who had recovered and (2) those who had not. These groupings were then arranged according to the following table of *observed frequencies* (Table 13.3).

It is immediately apparent from the table that more stutterers recovered ($N = 91$) than did not recover ($N = 21$); it is not known whether recovery can be attributed to therapy. Our null hypothesis of the χ^2 in this case will state the *observed frequencies* for the therapy group and the no-therapy group did not differ significantly from the *expected frequencies*, proportionate to the group as a whole.

Table 13.3. Data for the chi square.

Received Speech Therapy	Recovered		Totals
	Yes	No	
Yes	35	14	49
No	56	7	63
Totals	91	21	112

The expected frequencies are next determined by multiplying the two sub-totals from a given category, and dividing this result by the grand total.

$$f_e = \frac{(\text{sub-total } A)(\text{sub-total } B)}{\text{grand total}}$$

This computation may be illustrated from the previous table of observed frequencies (Table 13.4):

The rest of the expected frequencies, computed in the same manner are:

Received Therapy— Not Recovered	$\dfrac{(21)(49)}{112}$	=	$\dfrac{1029}{112}$	=	9.19
No Therapy— Recovered	$\dfrac{(91)(63)}{112}$	=	$\dfrac{5733}{112}$	=	51.19
No Therapy— Not Recovered	$\dfrac{(21)(63)}{112}$	=	$\dfrac{1323}{112}$	=	11.81

When both the observed frequencies (f_0) and the expected frequencies (f_e) are obtained, the work table for the χ^2 result may be set up (Table 13.5).

The resulting χ^2 of 5.5106 exceeds the value of 3.84 in the table of chi square, indicating a significance level of better than .05 for one degree of freedom. (Note: The value of 3.84 is always at the .05 level for all 2 × 2 chi squares.)

Table 13.4. Computation of the chi square.

Received Speech Therapy	Recovered		Totals B
	Yes	No	
Yes	35	14	49
No	56	7	63
Totals A	91	21	112

Expected Frequencies: f_e
Received Therapy- Recovered $\dfrac{(91)(49)}{112} \cong \dfrac{4459}{112} = 39.81$

Table 13.5. Work table for the chi square result.

Group	Observed Frequency f_0	Observed Frequency f_e	$f_0 - f_e$	$(f_0 - f_e)^2$	$\dfrac{(f_0 - f_e)^2}{f_e}$
Therapy- Recovered	35	39.81	−4.81	23.14	.5813
Therapy- Not Recovered	14	9.19	4.81	23.14	2.5180
No Therapy- Recovered	56	51.19	4.81	23.14	.4520
No Therapy- Not Recovered	7	11.81	−4.81	23.14	1.9593
Totals	112	112.00	0		$\chi^2 = 5.5106$

Degrees of freedom are determined by multiplying "rows-minus-one" by "columns-minus-one", as shown in the formula:

$$df = (\text{Rows-1})(\text{Columns-1})$$

$$df = (1)(1) = 1$$

This means that if we assign a frequency to one of the cells, the other three cells become automatically set. Therefore, the df in any 2×2 table is always equal to 1.

"Forced" Binomial Classification

A very useful application of the 2×2 chi square is one in which the data are not originally in the form of binomial tabulation but where the data have been classified as binomial on an a priori basis. This is sometimes called a *forced binomial classification*. It is usually made by a subjective evaluation of the data, according to scores which are "highest", and "lowest", "strongest", "weakest", etc., particularly when the data appear to be bimodal in distribution. This aspect of the scores may not be known until after the data are obtained and arranged. The dividing line for forced binomial classification is arbitrary, but it must be clearly explained in the results. If the number of scores is large, the comparison can be made between the upper third versus the lower third, with the middle third excluded. In other examples, the computation can be made by simply splitting the distribution into the upper half versus the lower half.

In an example of this type of data treatment, a survey of 86 recovered stutterers (Shearer and Williams, 1965) suggested that those who recovered normal speech at a younger age had less tendency for occasional nonfluency than did those who recovered at a much later age. For computation the subjects were divided into "early recovery" versus "late recovery." The "middle" recovery age was indecisive and was not used in the computation. Results of the chi square indicated that the consistency of eventual fluency was related to age of recovery.

THE X^2 FOR DATA HAVING MORE THAN TWO CATEGORIES

At times the data are not strictly binomial, but tend to fall into three or more categories, such as "small, medium, and large", "for, against, undecided", or might contain data from three or more groups, such as "student clinicians, school clinician, and supervising clinicians". As an example of this type of design, Sheehan and Williams, in the study mentioned earlier, wished to find whether recovery from stuttering was related to degree of severity in a group of 130 stutterers. Their data were arranged in Table 13.6:

Table 13.6. The 3×2 chi square.

Severity of Stuttering at Worst	Recovered		Totals
	Yes	No	
Mild	58	9	67
Moderate	35	12	47
Severe	8	8	16
Totals	101	29	130

Table 13.7. Results of the 3 × 2 chi square.

Group	Observed Frequency f_0	Expected Frequency f_e	$f_0 - f_e$	$(f_0 - f_e)^2$	$\dfrac{(f_0 - f_e)^2}{f_e}$
Mild-Recovered	58	52.05	5.95	35.40	.68
Mild-Not Recovered	9	14.95	−5.95	35.40	2.37
Moderate-Recovered	35	36.52	−1.52	2.31	.06
Moderate-Not Recovered	12	10.48	1.52	2.31	.22
Severe-Recovered	8	12.43	−4.43	19.62	1.58
Severe-Not Recovered	8	3.57	4.43	19.62	5.50
Totals	130				$\chi^2 = 10.41$

Although this illustrates a 2 × 3 table, the same computational procedure would apply if more categories were added to both variables.

The expected frequencies are derived in exactly the same manner as shown in the previous example, and the chi square may now be computed (Table 13.7).

The appropriate degrees of freedom, obtained by multiplying rows-minus-one, by columns-minus-one, is found to be 2.

$$df = (3 - 1)(2 - 1) = 2$$

The table of chi square indicates a critical value of 9.210 at the .01 probability. Sheehan's and Martyn's result of 10.41 exceeds this value, thereby rejecting the null hypothesis, and indicating that the result is significant.

CHAPTER 14

Computational
Exercises

Statistical Exercise 1: Choosing the statistic to fit the experimental design, and the type of data resulting from the measures.

For each of the following examples, write in the appropriate statistic from the matching list. Each statistic on the list should be selected for only one of the examples, based upon the criteria in the statistical selection chart in the section on choosing the appropriate statistic.

Matching List

t-test for independent measures
t-test for related measured
Treatments-by-subjects AOV
Treatments-by-groups AOV
One way AOV
Friedman's Test
Proportions Test

Wilcoxon Matched Pairs
Sign Test
Mann-Whitney U
Cochran Q
Spearman rho
Pearson r

Examples

1. Sheehan, J., Level of aspiration in female stutterers: changing times? *J. Speech Hearing Dis.*, 44, 479–486, 1979.
   Aspiration scores for a group of 21 female stutterers were compared with aspiration scores from a group of female nonstutterers. Data were considered to be normally distributed.
   Statistic: _____

2. Weiner, F., and Ostrowski, A., Effects of listener uncertainty on articulatory inconsistency. *J. Speech Hearing Dis.*, 44, 479–486, 1979.
   One group of 15 children was given articulation tests under 3 conditions. Scores were considered to be normally distributed.
   Statistic: _____

3. Hamre, C., and Wingate, M., Stuttering consistency in varied contexts. *J. Speech Hearing Res.*, 16, 238–247, 1973.
   The incidence of stuttering was compared according to 3 word positions in sentences (beginning, middle, or end) for a group of 16 stutterers. Stuttering incidence was rated in rank order for the 3 word positions.
   Statistic: _____

4. Lahey, M. Use of prosody and syntactic markers in children's comprehension of spoken sentences. *J. Speech Hearing Res.*, 17, 656–668, 1974.

Scores for four conditions of sentence presentation were compared for a group of nursery school children. Sentences were scored as either "correct" or "incorrect."
Statistic: _____

5. Wozniak, V., and Jackson, P., Visual vowel and diphthong perception from two horizontal viewing angles. *J. Speech Hearing Res.*, 22, 354–365, 1979.
The percentage of correctly perceived vowels was compared to the percentage of correctly perceived diphthongs, by one group of observers.
Statistic: _____

6. Kupperman, G., and Gengel, R., An argument for the use of a recorded speaker in the administration of a speech-in-noise test. *Language Speech Hearing Serv. Schools*, 10, 120–125, 1979.
Speech discrimination scores for 6 groups of subjects were compared. Each group contained 10 listeners, and data were considered normally distributed.
Statistic: _____

7. Silverman, E., The influence of preschooler's speech usage on their disfluency frequency. *J. Speech Hearing Res.*, 16, 474–483, 1973.
Fluency in one group of 10 normal-speaking four-year old boys was compared in two types of speech usage. Comparisons were scored as to which of the two usages had more disfluency (+) and which usage had less (−) disfluency for each subject.
Statistic: _____

8. Tweney, R., and Hoemann, H., The development of semantic associations in profoundly deaf children. *J. Speech Hearing Res.*, 16, 309–318, 1973.
Scores on a word-association test for a group of deaf children were compared with scores from a group of normal-hearing children. All scores were arranged in rank order for the comparison.
Statistic: _____

9. Tobey, E., Cullen, J., Rampp, D., and Fleischer-Gallagher, A., Effects of stimulus-onset asynchrony on the dichotic performance of children with auditory-processing disorders. *J. Speech Hearing Res.*, 22, 197–211, 1979.
A group of 8 auditory-disordered children and a group of 8 normal children were tested for speech perception accuracy under four dichotic listening conditions. Scores were normally distributed.
Statistic: _____

10. Sussman, H., Evidence for left hemisphere superiority in processing movement related tonal signals. *J. Speech Hearing Res.*, 22, 224–235, 1979.
As part of the study one group of subjects was tested for right ear tone-tracking accuracy, compared with left ear tone-tracking accuracy. The two sets of laterality scores were not treated as normally distributed data.
Statistic: _____

11. Shewan, C., and Kertesz, A., Reliability and validity characteristics of the Western Aphasia Battery (WAB). *J. Speech Hearing Dis.*, 45, 308–324, 1980.
Subtests on the Western Aphasia Battery were re-administered to a sample of 38 aphasic patients, to establish a test-retest correlation for reliability.
Statistic: _____

12. McGlone, R., and Shipp, T., Some physiologic correlates of vocal-fry phonation. *J. Speech Hearing Res.*, 14, 769–775, 1971.

Airflow measures during vocal fry and modal phonation were compared from a group of 9 subjects. Data were normally distributed.
Statistic: _____

13. Needham, L., and Swisher, L., A comparison of three tests of auditory comprehension for adult aphasics. *J. Speech Hearing Dis.*, 37, 123–131, 1972. Part of the study analyzed the relationship between scores on two types of tests, to determine how well the score from one test would predict the score on another. Scores for each analysis were arranged in rank order.
Statistic: _____

COMPUTATIONAL EXERCISE 2: *t*-TEST FOR INDEPENDENT MEASURES

Examples

Sussman, H., Evidence for left hemisphere superiority in processing moment related tonal signals. *J. Speech Hearing Res.*, 22, 224–335, 1979.
Scores from subjects receiving binaural auditory cues were compared with those receiving monaural auditory cues.

Shapiro, I., Evaluation of the relationship between hearing threshold and loudness discomfort level in sensorineural hearing loss. *J. Speech Hearing Dis.*, 44, 31–36, 1979.
Loudness discomfort levels for the severe hearing loss group were compared to those for the moderate hearing loss group.

Rucello, D., and Shelton, R., Planning and self assessment in articulation training. *J. Speech Hearing Dis.*, 44, 504–512, 1979.
Articulation improvements from two groups of children were compared: those who planned their performance in advance, and those who did not plan.

Computational Data

Select a comparison of two groups from one of the t-test examples and write the group names above the sample data.

Table 14.1. Data for the computation of t.

Group 1	Group 2
5	1
6	2
7	3
7	3
7	3
8	4
9	6

Total $\Sigma X =$
Mean $\bar{X} =$
Number of scores $N =$
df =

COMPUTATIONAL EXERCISE 3: MANN-WHITNEY U

Examples

Ingham, R., and Packman, A., Perceptual assessment of normalcy of speech following stuttering therapy. *J. Speech Hearing Res.*, 21, 63–73, 1978.

One part of the study compared listener judgement scale data for two speaker groups: fluent speech from stutterers and from normal speakers.

Hess, D., A new experimental approach to assessment of velopharyngeal adequacy: nasal manometric bleed testing. *J. Speech Hearing Dis.*, 41, 427–443, 1976.

Manometric measures for cleft palate and normal speakers were compared.

Leonard, L., Miller, J., and Brown, H., Consonant and syllable harmony in the speech of language-disordered children. *J. Speech Hearing Dis.*, 45, 336–345, 1980.

Instances of reduplication of syllables were compared in two groups of language-disordered children.

Computational Data

Select one of the examples for computation and write in the names of the two groups at the top of the data samples.

Table 14.2. Data for the computation of U. Scores from two independent groups of subjects.

Group 1	Group 2
0.0	2.0
.6	5.1
3.2	6.9
4.0	8.2
7.3	8.8
	9.1
	9.2
	9.5
	9.9
Σ Ranks 1 =	Σ Ranks 2 =
N_1 =	N_2 =

COMPUTATIONAL EXERCISE 4: PROPORTIONS TEST z

Examples

Silliman, E., Relationship between pictorial interpretation and comprehension of three special relations in school age children. *J. Speech Hearing Res.*, 22, 366–388, 1979.

The proportion of comprehension for the concept "in back of" was compared with comprehension for "in front of."

Eilers, R., Wilson, W., and Moore, J., Development changes in speech discrimination in infants. *J. Speech Hearing Res.*, 20, 766–780, 1977.

One part of the study compared the proportion of infants' responses to hearing a change in syllables as compared to the same syllable repeated.

Carpenter, R., and Rutherford, D. Acoustic cue discrimination in adult aphasia. *J. Speech Hearing Res.*, 16, 534–544, 1973.

The proportion of aphasics who passed an auditory discrimination test was compared with the proportion of the normal control group who passed the same test.

Computational Data

Select one of the examples for computation and write the names representing the two proportions in the title spaces.

	Proportion 1	Proportion 2
Total observations:	$N_1 = 200$	$N_2 = 140$
Total positive score:	$X_1 = 180$	$X_2 = 70$
Group proportion:	$P_1 = \dfrac{X_1}{N_1} = .\underline{\hspace{1cm}}$	$P_2 = .\underline{\hspace{1cm}}$

COMPUTATIONAL EXERCISE 5: *t*-TEST FOR RELATED MEASURES

Examples

Wismer, G., and Ingrisano, D., Phrase-level timing patterns in English: emphatic stress location and reading rate. *J. Speech Hearing Res.*, 22, 516–553, 1979.

Duration of emphasized words was compared with nonemphasized words, using one group of subjects.

Tannahill, J., The hearing handicap scale as a measure of hearing aid benefit. *J. Speech Hearing Dis.*, 44, 91–99, 1979.

Speech reception thresholds with hearing aids were compared with unaided thresholds.

Bowman, S., and Shanks, J., Velopharyngeal relationships of /i/ and /s/ as seen cephalemetrically for persons with suspected incompetance. *J. Speech Hearing Dis.*, 43, 185–191, 1978.

Velopharyngeal gap for /i/ was compared with a gap shown for /s/ in one group of subjects.

Computational Data

Select one of the examples for computation and write the names of the two measures at the top of the data samples.

Table 14.3. Data for the computation of t.

Subjects	Measure 1 Title: _____	Measure 2 Title: _____
1	1	3
2	2	4
3	3	6
4	3	6
5	3	6
6	4	8
7	5	9
Totals	$\Sigma X_1 =$	$\Sigma X_2 =$
Means	$\bar{X}_1 =$	$\bar{X}_2 =$
N =		
df =		
t =		

COMPUTATIONAL EXERCISE 6: WILCOXON MATCHED PAIRS *T*

Examples

Mowrer, D., and Scoville, A., Response bias in children's phonological systems. *J. Speech Hearing Dis.*, 43, 473–481, 1978.
As one part of the study the imitative responses from a group of children were compared for accuracy of initial and final consonants.

Brutten, G., and Janssen, P., An eye-marking investigation of anticipated and observed stuttering. *J. Speech Hearing Res.*, 22, 20–26, 1979.
Comparisons of eye fixation were made before stuttered and nonstuttered words.

Sussman, H., Evidence for left hemisphere superiority in processing movement related tonal signals. *J. Speech Hearing Res.*, 22 224–235, 1979.
The study compared tracking accuracy scores for left ear signals and right ear signals, for one group of subjects.

Computational Data

Select one of the examples for computation and write the names of the two measures at the top of the data samples.

Table 14.4. Data for the computation of T.

Subjects	Measure 1	Measure 2	Difference (+ or −)	Rank of Difference	Less Frequent Sign Ranks
1	10	14			
2	11	17			
3	12	17			
4	13	11			
5	17	26			
6	19	27			
7	20	23			
8	20	19			

N =   T =
                                                        Significance level =

COMPUTATIONAL EXERCISE 7: SIGN TEST z

Examples

Smith, B., Weinberg, B., Feth, L., and Horii, Y., Vocal roughness and jitter characteristics of vowels produced by esophageal speakers *J. Speech Hearing Res.*, 21, 240–249, 1978.

Listeners judged relative vocal roughness in pairs of vowels.

Johns, D., and Darley, F., Phonemic variability in apraxia of speech. *J. Speech Hearing Res.*, 13, 556–583, 1970.

One part of the study compared accuracy of perception for a list of real words with perception of nonsense words.

Tillman, T., Carhart, R., and Olsen, W., Hearing aid efficiency in a competing speech situation. *J. Speech Hearing Res.*, 13, 789–811, 1970.

Various samples of aided and unaided speech discrimination scores were compared.

Computational Data

Select one of the examples for computation and write in the names of the two groups at the top of the data samples. Note: Tied scores are omitted from the computation.

Table 14.5. Data for the computation of z.

Set 1		Set 2	Direction of the Difference
1		2	
1		3	
2		3	
2		1	
2		3	
1		3	
1		2	
2		3	
1		2	
3	(tie)	3	

$$z =$$
Significance =

COMPUTATIONAL EXERCISE 8: BINOMIAL TEST *z*

Oller, D., Payne, S., and Gavin, W., Tactual speech perception by minimally trained deaf subjects. *J. Speech Hearing Res.*, 23, 769–778, 1980.

Subjects were shown a choice of two words to respond to each tactual presentation. One of the words shown was the correct choice and the other was incorrect, allowing a chance score of 50%.

Cooper, M., and Allen, G., Timing control accuracy in normal speakers and stutterers. *J. Speech Hearing Res.*, 20, 55–71, 1977.

Long reading durations were tabulated for paragraphs read early in the sequence, compared to paragraphs read late in the sequence. The Binomial Test was used to evaluate the proportion of long durations for the early paragraphs.

Computational Exercise

Observed score = 25
Number of total items = 40

$$z = \frac{\rule{3cm}{0.4pt}}{\sqrt{\rule{3cm}{0pt}}}$$

COMPUTATIONAL EXERCISE 9:
ONE WAY ANALYSIS OF VARIANCE

Examples

Murry, T., Speaking fundamental frequency characteristics associated with
voice pathologies. *J. Speech Hearing Dis.*, 43, 374–379, 1978.
The study compared fundamental frequency for normal voices and various
vocal pathologies.

Yorkston, K., and Beukelman, D., An analysis of connected speech samples
of asphasic and normal speakers. *J. Speech Hearing Dis.*, 45, 27–36, 1980.
The analysis included normals, geriatrics, and three different severity
groups of aphasics.

Silman, S. and Gelfand, S., Prediction of hearing levels from acoustic reflex
thresholds in persons with high frequency hearing loss. *J. Speech Hearing
Res.*, 22, 697–707, 1979.
One part of the study compared the mean acoustic reflex thresholds of one
normal group and three hearing loss groups.

Computational Data

Select three group titles from one of the examples.

Table 14.6. Data for the computation of F.

Group 1	Group 2	Group 3
1	3	6
3	4	7
3	4	7
3	4	7
4	5	8

Totals ΣX
Means $\bar{X}$
Total Squared
Scores ΣX^2
Subjects per group =   Number of groups =

COMPUTATIONAL EXERCISE 10: KRUSKAL-WALLIS *H*

Examples

Sarno, M., Silverman, M., and Sands, E., Speech therapy and language recovery in severe aphasia. *J. Speech Hearing Res.*, 13, 607–623, 1970.
Programmed instruction, non-programmed instruction and no-treatment groups were compared. H test was significant, with non-programmed therapy group diplaying highest performance in some areas.

Ritterman, S., The role of practice and observation of practice in speech sound discrimination learning. *J. Speech Hearing Res.*, 13, 178–183, 1970.
Practice, observation of practice and no-practice groups were compared. H test was significant, with the no-practice group showing the lowest scores.

Computational Data

Select three group titles from one of the examples.

Table 14.7. Data for the computation of H.

Group 1	Group 2	Group 3
26	29	43
30	32	52
16	40	60
20	38	47
18	31	39

Total Ranks ΣR =
Total Ranks Squared $(\Sigma R)^2$ =
Total Subjects =

COMPUTATIONAL EXERCISE 11: TREATMENTS-BY-SUBJECTS ANALYSIS OF VARIANCE *F*

Examples

Horii, Y., Vocal shimmer in sustained phonation. *J. Speech Hearing Res.*, 23, 202–209, 1980.

Vocal shimmer measures were compared for three vowel productions (/i/, /a/, and /u/) from one group of subjects.

Millen, C., and Prutting, C., Inconsistencies across three language comprehension tests for specific grammatical features. *Language Speech Hearing Serv. Schools*, 10, 162–170, 1979.

One part of the study compared mean performance, using the same subject's scores on three language tests.

Reich, A., and Lerman, J., Teflon pharyngoplasty: an acoustical and perceptual study. *J. Speech Hearing Dis.*, 43, 496–505, 1978.

Means of judges' ratings for hoarseness were compared at pre-treatment and after several post-treatment intervals.

Computational Data

Write in three group titles from one of the examples.

Table 14.8. Data for the computation of F.

Group 1	Group 2	Group 3
1	5	7
3	8	6
5	7	7
2	6	9
3	7	8

Total $\Sigma X =$
Mean $\bar{X} =$
Number of Subjects $N =$ Number of Groups =

COMPUTATIONAL EXERCISE 12: FRIEDMAN TEST χ^2

Examples

Bliss, L., Guilford, A., and Tikofsky, R., Performance of adult aphasics in a sentence evaluation and revision task. *J. Speech Hearing Res.*, 19, 536–550, 1976.

Numbers of correct evaluations made by a group of aphasics were compared for several types of sentences.

Carroll, J. and Tanenhaus, M., Functional clauses and sentence segmentation. *J. Speech Hearing Res.*, 21, 793–808, 1978.

Listeners' accuracy in marking the location of a tone in four types of clausal sentences was evaluated. Results showed listeners' tendency to perceive the tones as being located at the boundaries of functionally complete clauses.

Mowrer, D., Wahl, P., and Doolan, S., Effect of lisping on audience evaluation of male speakers. *J. Speech Hearing Res.*, 43, 140–148, 1978.

Listeners rated a number of adult speakers according to a scale of personal characteristics. Lispers were rated significantly lower than nonlispers.

Computational Data

Write in four group titles from one of the examples.

Table 14.9. Data for Friedman's χ^2.

Group 1	Group 2	Group 3	Group 4
1	2	3	4
2	1	3	4
1	3	2	4
1	2	4	3
1	2	3	4

Total Ranks $\Sigma R =$
Squared total $(\Sigma R)^2 =$
Sum of Squared Ranks $\Sigma(R^2) =$

COMPUTATIONAL EXERCISE 13: COCHRAN Q TEST

Examples

Lahey, W., Use of prosody and syntactic markers in children's comprehension of spoken sentences. *J. Speech Hearing Res.*, 17, 656–668, 1974.

The Q test was used to compare the correct-incorrect responses from a group of children to sentences presented under several different conditions.

Thurlow, W., and Jacques, J., Localization of two noise sources overlapping in time. *J. Speech Hearing Res.*, 18, 653–662, 1975.

One part of the study compared accuracy of discriminating one versus two sounds, using several different onset intervals between the pairs of sounds.

Block, J., and Gersten, E., and Kornblum, S., Evaluation of a language program for young autistic children. *J Speech Hearing Dis.*, 45, 76–89, 1980.

A group of autistic children were tested for gains in several behavioral categories over a two year period. Some of the more significant categories included vocal play, vocal imitation, and expressive speech.

Computational Data

Fill in the names of three test categories from one of the examples.

Table 14.10. Data for the computation of Q

Category 1	Category 2	Category 3
+	+	−
−	+	−
+	+	−
+	−	−
+	−	+
+	+	−
+	+	−
+	+	−
+	−	−
+	−	−

Total Minus Scores
Totals Squared
Grand Total =   Sum of All Totals Squared =   Sum of Subject Totals Squared =

COMPUTATIONAL EXERCISE 14: TREATMENTS-BY-GROUPS

(Two factor analysis of variance with repeated measures on one factor)

Examples

Haynes, W., Purcell, E., and Haynes, M., A pragmatic aspect of language sampling. *Language Speech Hearing Serv. Schools*, 10, 104–110, 1979.
Results compared MLU scores for 4 and 6 year old children tested under three conditions.

Panagos, J., and King, R., Self and mutual speech comprehension by deviant and normal-speaking children. *J. Speech Hearing Res.*, 18, 634–652, 1975.
Comprehension scores from two groups of children (normal and deviant-speaking) were compared for different types of sentences.

Nelson, L., and Weber-Olsen, M., The elicited language inventory and the influence of contextual cues, *J. Speech Hearing Dis.*, 45, 549–563, 1980.
Scores from the Elicited Language Inventory (ELI) were compared for two groups of children (normal and language delayed) under different conditions of presentation.

Computational Data

Write in the titles of the groups and treatments from one of the referenced examples.

Table 14.11. Data for the computation of F.

	Test 1		Test 2		Test 3	
	X	X^2	X	X^2	X	X^2
Group 1	1		2		5	
	3		3		6	
	3		3		6	
	3		3		6	
	5		5		7	
Group 2	2		3		6	
	3		4		7	
	3		4		7	
	3		4		7	
	4		5		8	

Total $\Sigma X =$
Total Squared $(\Sigma X)^2 =$
Total Squared Scores $\Sigma(X^2) =$

COMPUTATIONAL EXERCISE 15: TREATMENTS-BY-TREATMENTS-BY-SUBJECTS ANALYSIS OF VARIANCE

Examples

Young, L., Goodman, J., and Carhart, R., The intelligibility of whitened and amplitude compressed speech in a multitalker background. *J. Speech Hearing Res.*, 23, 383–392, 1980.

This study compared scores from one group of subjects for different modes of speech processing and different signal-to-noise ratios.

Sorensen, D., Horii, Y., and Leonard, R., Effects of laryngeal topical anesthesia on voice fundamental frequency perturbation. *J. Speech Hearing Res.*, 23, 274–283, 1980.

Different fundamental frequencies were compared with and without anesthesia for one group of subjects. Scores were in the form of vocal jitter measures.

Computational Data

Write in the headings for factor A and factor B from one of the examples. In factor B each category is shown twice.

Table 14.12. Data for the computation of F.

Factor A	————		————	
Factor B	————	————	————	————
1	1	5	4	7
2	3	8	8	6
3	5	7	7	7
4	2	6	6	9
5	3	7	7	8

Total $\Sigma X =$
Total Squared $(\Sigma X)^2 =$
Squared Scores $\Sigma(X^2) =$

COMPUTATIONAL EXERCISE 16:
TUKEY TEST FOR POST HOC ANALYSIS

Examples

Thompson, D., Sills, J., Recke, K., and Bui, D., Acoustic reflex growth in the aging adult. *J. Speech Hearing Res.*, 23, 393–404, 1980.

As one part of the study, reflex thresholds from several different audiometric frequencies were compared by the Tukey test, following analysis of variance.

Iglesias, A., Kuehn, D., and Morris, H., Simultaneous assessment of pharyngeal wall and velar displacement for selected speech sounds. *J. Speech Hearing Res.*, 23, 429–446, 1980.

Velar displacements for several different phonemes were compared by the Tukey test following analysis for variance.

Scott, C., and Taylor A., A comparison of home and clinic gathered language samples. *J. Speech Hearing Dis.*, 43, 482–495, 1978.

The Tukey test compared mean length of utterances for speech samples in various settings.

Computational Data

Table 14.13. Source table for the analysis of variance.

Source	Sums of Squares	df	Mean Squares	F
Between Groups	50.0	2	25.0	
Within Groups	18.0	9	2.0	12.50
(Error Term)				

Group 1 Mean = 12.25   Subjects per group = 10
Group 2 Mean = 17.50 q Probability = .05
Group 3 Mean = 24.75
q value =
Standard Error =
Critical Difference =

COMPUTATIONAL EXERCISE 17: SCHEFFÉ TEST FOR POST HOC ANALYSIS

Examples

Haynes, W., Purcell, E., and Haynes, M., A pragmatic aspect of language sampling. *Language Speech Hearing Serv. Schools*, 10, 104–110, 1979.

Differences in language (DSS) scores from several types of language sampling techniques were compared by the Scheffé test following a significant F result.

Ruscello, D., Lass, N., Fultz, N., and Hug, M., Attitudes of educators toward speech-language pathology services in rural schools. *Language Speech Hearing Serv. Schools*, 11, 139–144, 1980.

Attitudes of educators toward several types of school programs (including speech-language therapy) were evaluated by rating questionnaire scores. Differences between specific ratings were determined by the Scheffé following significant analysis of variance.

Cohill, E., and Greenberg, H., Effects of ethyl alcohol on the contralateral and ipsilateral acoustic reflex threshold. *J. Speech Hearing Res.*, 22, 289–294, 1979.

Scheffé test was used to compare differences in acoustic reflex thresholds under several levels of blood-alcohol concentrations.

Computational Data

Table 14.14. Source for the analysis of variance.

Source	Sums of Squares	df	Mean Squares	F
Between Groups	50.0	2	25.0	
Within Groups (Error Term)	18.0	9	2.0	12.50

Group 1 Mean = 12.25	Subjects per group = 10
Group 2 Mean = 17.50	Number of Groups = 3
Group 3 Mean = 24.75	F Factor Probability = .05

COMPUTATIONAL EXERCISE 18: NEWMAN-KUELS TEST FOR POST HOC ANALYSIS

Examples

Yorkston, K., and Beukelman, D., An analysis of connected speech samples of aphasic and normal speakers. *J. Speech Hearing Dis.*, 45, 27–36, 1980.

One part of the post hoc testing revealed that speaking rates for normal adults and geriatric adults were significantly higher than those of the aphasic speakers.

Moore, W., and Haynes, W., Alpha hemispheric asymmetry and stuttering: some support for a segmentation dysfunction hypothesis. *J. Speech Hearing Res.*, 23, 229–247, 1980.

One part of the post hoc testing revealed greater alpha wave activity for the right hemisphere during verbal tasks for the normal females and males than for stutterers.

Kupperman, G., and Gengel, R., An argument for the use of a recorded speaker in the administration of a speech-in-noise test. *Language Speech Hearing Serv. Schools*, 10, 120–125, 1979.

Post hoc testing revealed significant differences among speech discrimination tests administered by different speakers in the presence of a standardized noise.

Computational Data

Table 14.15. Source table for the analysis of variance.

Source	Sums of Squares	df	Mean Squares	F
Between Groups	50.0	2	25.0	12.50
Within Groups (Error Term)	18.0	9	2.0	

Group A Mean = 12.25   Subjects per group = 10
Group B Mean = 17.50   Range of Ranks for three groups:
Group C Mean = 24.75   A − B =
                               A − C =
                               B − C =
                               Probability for q = .05

COMPUTATIONAL EXERCISE 19:
PEARSON COEFFICIENT OF COORELATION *r*

Examples

Gerken, K., Language Dominance: a comparison of measures. *Language Speech Hearing Serv. Schools*, 9, 187–196, 1978.
    Correlations were made for the scores of 32 Mexican-American children on English and Spanish versions of verbal tests.
Fletcher, S., and Higgins, J., Performance of children with severe to profound auditory impairment in instrumentally guided reduction of nasal resonance. *J. Speech Hearing Dis.*, 45, 181–194, 1980.
    Correlations were computed between percentage of nasal resonance and number of training sessions.
Shewan, C., and Kertesz, A., Reliability and validity characteristics of the Western Aphasia Battery (WAB). *J. Speech Hearing Dis.*, 45, 308–324, 1980.
    Test-retest reliability of subtest scores were evaluated by r correlations.

Computational Data

Write in the titles of two groups of data from one of the examples.

Table 14.16. Data for the computation of *r*.

Group 1		Group 2		
X	X^2	Y	Y^2	XY
1		3		
3		5		
3		4		
4		5		
5		6		
6		7		
7		6		
7		7		
7		8		
8		8		
9		10		
10		9		
11		12		
11		12		
12		11		
Totals =				

COMPUTATIONAL EXERCISE 20: SPEARMAN RHO

Examples

Coleman, R., A comparison of the contributions of two voice quality characteristics to the perception of maleness and femaleness in the voice. *J. Speech Hearing Res.*, 19, 168–180, 1976.

Rank orders of fundamental frequency and male-female voice quality were evaluated by means of the Spearman rho.

Dworkin, J., Characteristics of frontal lispers clustered according to severity. *J. Speech Hearing Dis.*, 45, 37–44, 1980.

One part of the study tested for the relationship between relative severity of lisping and length of tongue.

Erber, N., and Alencewicz, C., Audiologic evaluation of deaf children. *J. Speech Hearing Dis.*, 41, 256–267, 1976.

Part of the study was to consider the rank order correlation for degree of cerumen occlusion in the ear canals, as rated by the audiologist and by the pediatrician.

Computational Data

Write in the name of the two measures or types of rating used in one of the examples of Spearman rho data analysis.

Table 14.17. Data for the computation of rho.

Measure 1		Measure 2			
	Ranking 1		Ranking 2	Difference	Difference^2
1		101			
2		100			
3		102			
4		104			
5		105			
6		103			
7		106			
8		107			
9		108			
10		111			
11		109			
12		110			

Total Squared Differences $\sum D^2$

COMPUTATIONAL EXERCISES 21: TWO-BY-TWO CHI SQUARE χ^2

Examples

Richman, L., Cognitive patterns and learning disabilities in cleft palate children with verbal deficits. *J. Speech Hearing Res.*, 23, 429–446, 1980.
  The study tested the relationship for two classifications of cleft palate with two levels of language disability.

Silvestri, S., and Sylvestri, R., A developmental analysis of the acquisition of compound words. *Lang. Speech Hearing Serv. Schools*, 8, 217–221, 1977.
  A chi square was used to study the relationship between two children's grade levels and two levels of the children's verbal responses.

Fisher, L., Efficiency and effectiveness of using a portable audiometric booth in school hearing conservation programs. *Lang. Speech Hearing Serv. Schools*, 7, 242–249, 1976.
  Chi square was used to observed the presence-absence of hearing loss found in persons tested in two types of testing situations.

Computational Data

Fill in the two categories under classification A and the two categories of classification B for the observed values in the chi square table.

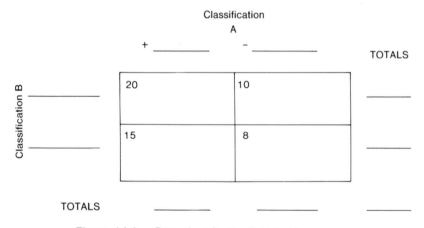

Figure 14.1.   Data chart for the 2 × 2 chi square.

PART 3

Research Writing

CHAPTER 15 Research Writing

The writing of research reports, such as articles, dissertations, convention papers, theses, and term papers, requires a style which is rather formal but which conveys the information clearly and effectively to the reader. Good research is not always synonymous with good writing, and some of our most respected researchers are actually quite poor journalists. An article which is stilted, encumbered by nonessential detail, and which over-qualifies the essential points does not communicate well with the reader. Although scholarly in appearance, this type of writing style should not be the student's goal. Any article which must be read three times in order to be understood is not written for the reader.

In the process of developing one's writing style it is important to note that good prose need not be stuffy; it can even be somewhat conversational, as in:

"There are several problems in acoustic phonetics that could be answered at least partially if it were possible to get clear spectrograms from children's voices."

(Huggins, 1980, p. 19)

Although vocabulary may be relatively formal, the sentence can be simple, clear, and to the point:

"One consistent characteristic of children with severe mental retardation is extremely delayed language development."

(Eilers and Oller, 1980, p. 425)

Paradoxically, the writing utilized in our graduate training programs is not always consistent with the writing which is later to become a part of one's professional career. The achievement of effective writing style is therefore complicated by the difference in expectations for each type of setting. The tedious detail and extensive review of the literature expected for the dissertation or thesis is in sharp contrast to the brevity and efficiency needed for an acceptable journal article. While graduate training in research is to foster thoroughness and complete consideration of all major and minor points, the journal editor must be concerned with page limitations and brevity as well as quality. Through this paradox, the author of an admirable dissertation or thesis may find his first article rejected because his meticulous descriptions appear as amateurish trivia in the journal manuscript. Much to their credit, some training programs encourage the completion of a journal article in addition to the standard graduate paper, in order to make this critical transition in professional research writing.

INITIATING THE WRITING PROJECT

In addition to developing technique and craftsmanship for professional writing the sheer act of starting the written work and seeing it through to the finish constitutes a major—sometimes awesome—step which has received virtually no attention. The often-heard comment, "My research was finished last year; I just haven't written the dissertation yet", is a testament to the seriousness of the student's problem. Nor is the faculty immune to similar procrastination; the old saw, "I've got three in the drawer", is a sad commentary to unwritten research.

There are no limits to the reasons why some studies are conducted up to the point of the written report, only to lie dormant at the threshold of completion. In some cases, it may be that once the study itself is completed the writing is an anticlimax, which comes at a time when the work should have ended. For others, a disenchantment in the topic or a disappointment in the results may contribute to lack of motivation in its writing phase. Regardless of contributing factors, however, a fundamental core to the problem seems to be in the tiresome prospect of sitting down to a typewriter and facing a blank sheet of paper. Those who write on a fairly regular basis have developed a number of tricks or strategies to get moving ahead with the chore. One journalism professor advised his student to, "place your fingers on the typewriter keys and simply start them moving. Don't try to think of the words yourself; let the typewriter do the thinking for you." Strange though it may sound, this transfer of responsibility to the typewriter's keys reduces the writing effort. Apparently it is easier to think of ideas than to think of words. After a few practice sessions, the rough draft produced by this method can provide a reliable basis for the eventual finished manuscript.

A similar method in getting the manuscript started is based upon an old principle of general semantics, wherein one sits at the typewriter and concentrates on a steady and creative flow of ideas. If the flow does not occur it suggests that the writer is too tense, is trying too hard, or is expecting too much perfection for the first draft. The flow of ideas is essentially a mental set toward relaxation. The basic principle is not to restrict or censor the words as they develop on the page, and to ignore one's compulsions and perfectionistic tendencies until the later editing of the manuscript. Any thoughts which come to mind should be written immediately and spontaneously. Once this technique is developed, it can produce a good start on a difficult topic.

A final technique, which we might call the "study hall approach to research writing", requires that the writer sit at the typewriter for a prescribed period of time at the same hour each day. The time period should be relatively short—between 20 minutes and one hour—and the only rule is that it must be carried out every day with no exceptions or excuses. Some sessions will hardly be worth the trouble, adding only a few belabored lines to the page, but others will go considerably beyond expectations. Progress by this method is based upon average progress over many sessions rather than the success of any one sitting.

All of these methods have a common goal: to over-ride one's natural sedentary inertia and to transform good intentions into productive behavior. Regardless of the method employed to develop the manuscript, some additional guidance and reference to examples is needed by the inexperienced writer to help in the use of terminology and in achieving the sense of efficiency and accuracy needed in good research journalism. The sections which follow have been used effectively in helping students in their initial stages of research writing. A number of examples are presented to assist the student in developing his own prose and to reduce the amount of editing required from his advisor.

In its conceptual form, the research report is in the nature of an argument. The researcher takes the view that he or she has found something valid and worth reporting, and the reader takes the role of skeptic or critic, who is not necessarily convinced that the researcher's findings are really well founded or worthwhile. In many respects, this classical role of research presentation is in the realm of theory or research philosophy, but it may be taken quite literally at any time. This is illustrated dramatically when the results of a convention paper are abruptly and unexpectedly challenged, or when an article is criticized in a letter to the editor. The vulnerability to criticism is a constant reminder to the researcher that his claims must be able to withstand critical scrutiny. To publish research is to invite a challenge, which may be one reason why some who are capable scholars are reluctant to publish their work. Nearly every journal contains an example of this type of challenge:

"We are responding to this article not because we find fault with the author's data but because we object to the premise that lateral cephalometry provides a valid diagnostic tool for assessing the velopharyngeal sphincter."

(Glaser *et al.*, 1979, p. 557)

Criticism from the editors of refereed journals may be less polite. The following excerpts are from colleagues' anonymous reviews of manuscripts sent to journals for consideration toward publication:

"Although the manuscript is fraught with split infinitives and contributes little beyond what is already known, I recommend that it be accepted for publication because of the popular interest in this topic."

In some instances, the anonymous reviewer's comments appear more as an insult than a critique:

"I suggest that the manuscript be refused for publication, and in view of the author's incompetence, further work on the manuscript should not be encouraged."

The student who intends to continue his or her scholarship into professional life must realize that criticism is a natural part of the game. It does not end when the thesis is completed; it is just the beginning. Criticism is a healthy and necessary part of objectivity.

In view of the preceeding discussion, some valuable insights into research writing are easily made. The researcher must be able to read his own work from the viewpoint of the critic or the disbeliever or to ask someone else to probe for flaws in the manuscript. An encouraging and supportive friend is not always the best person to choose if honest criticism is needed.

The written report must include enough information to convince the reader that all the necessary precautions were taken in the procedure, that the results were correctly derived from the statistics, and that the implications and conclusions are realistic and based upon a solid foundation. Each part of the written work must be viewed, in the final analysis, as a part of the overall convincing argument.

OUTLINE OF THE THESIS AND DISSERTATION

In the thesis, dissertation, article, or convention paper the sequence of informational presentation is nearly always the same, but it should be emphasized that a five chapter outline is by no means the only appropriate format. In some examples of research works the selection of subjects, the instrumentation, or the test materials may require greater description so as to demand the addition of another chapter or section in the thesis. In other instances, the results and discussion chapters may be combined, or the introduction and review of the literature might similarly be presented as one chapter instead of two. In the journal article, where brevity is a prime consideration of the editor, the review of the literature is nearly always omitted as a separate section.

In summary, the majority of theses and dissertations are set up as five chapters, but some may have only a four chapter format and a few may include as many as six or seven.

The outline which follows is intended only as a general guide to the content of each chapter. It may easily be modified according to the needs of the investigation at hand. Discussion and examples of the major points in this outline follow in the succeeding chapter headings.

I. Introduction
    a. The importance of, or interest in the research topic
    b. Directly related investigations, parallel studies, or commentary which serve as immediate background
    c. Inadequacy of present information about the topic, due to limitations in previous studies or a general lack of investigation
    d. Ways in which the present study intends to overcome previous deficiencies or to add new information
    e. The specifically stated purpose or hypotheses of the present study

II. Review of the Literature
    a. Preparatory comments about the literature, including subtopics, limitations, problems, or special considerations.
    b. Presentation of the most closely related studies, in which the most significant ones may be summarized in some detail
    c. Studies farther removed from the present study are included as needed to provide depth and scope to the research topic

III. Method
    a. Description of the subjects
    b. Description of the instrumentation, which may include diagrams if new or unusual equipment is used
    c. Measuring techniques, tests, and reliability procedures
    d. Arrangments used in the gathering, grouping, and analysis of data

IV. Results
    a. Statistical treatment and numerical results
    b. Verbal statement of each result as it relates to the hypothesis
    c. Supplementary statement as to agreement or disagreement with previous studies
    d. Charts or graphic display which might be needed to summarize trends or other features of the results

V. Discussion
    a. Implications of the results as they relate to the questions or problems raised in the introduction
    b. Considerations of the strengths or weaknesses of the present study, if applicable

c. Tentative hypotheses and suggestions for continued or related new research in the same general area

THE INTRODUCTION

Here the reader is presented with some information to familiarize him with the topic, and the reason for the research project is explained. The purpose of the study may be in the nature of substantiating clinical observations, shedding light on some theoretical concept, or taking issue for or against a previous study. Ideally, the introduction should also cite one or more references upon which the study is based. Further, it should be shown in what way previous research in the area of interest is nonexistent, incomplete, or otherwise inadequate. Overall, the introduction should include the logic for the project's inception—in a way, an argument to justify the research endeavor.

A well written introduction should begin with a strong informative statement which will lead the reader directly into the topic. The lead statement preferably should catch the reader's attention with a concise picture of the main point of the research. Many reports unfortunately begin with a neutral filler sentence, such as, "Audiologists have long been concerned with the problem of hearing loss." This sentence says essentially nothing, and puts the reader no farther into the topic. In contrast, a sentence such as, "A matter of critical concern for the audiologist is in the reasons why a recommended hearing aid is not worn by the potential user", brings the reader directly to the heart of the study.

The first paragraph should supply the most essential background information to show where the study fits into the overall body of knowledge surrounding the topic, so that the reader can see that the study is the next logical step in the continuing development of knowledge. A poorly written introduction in the thesis may lead the reader on for several pages before finally revealing the purpose of the study. It is difficult, if not impossible, for the reader to associate the information unless the central theme is revealed right from the beginning. Once the aim of the study and the place where the study is to fit into the literature is shown, more general or remote background may be introduced, which may refer to the history or the diversity of the topic. This type of information serves to enrich the oncept, and is added to furnish a more complete picture.

With a less experienced writer it is not unusual to find a good lead paragraph near the middle or end of the introduction, rather than at the beginning. Some forms of writing are intended to build the theme gradually so as to arouse curiosity or to develop the plot, but this approach is more appropriate for the mystery story than for the research report. The thesis or dissertation should be viewed more as an informative article than as an essay, although it may contain elements of both.

The end of the introduction should refer specifically to the questions to be answered or to the hypothesis to be tested by the research method. The more specifically these points are stated, the better the reader will know exactly what to look for in the results section of the report. For clarity in the thesis or dissertation the points to be tested should best be designated by numerical order, while the journal article is more inclined to refer to a general summarizing statement of the hypothesis.

These elements of the study may appear as:

Specifically, the present study was designed to answer the following three questions:

1. Is there a difference between the vocabulary test scores for 5-year-old children and 6-year-old children?
2. Is there a difference between the compound verb usage of 5-year-old children and 6-year-old children?
3. Is there a difference in vocabulary and verb usage scores for 5 and 6-year-old inner city children as compared with children of the same age attending suburban schools?

In its abbreviated journal style, the same material would read:

The present investigation was designed to study two language categories of 5 and 6-year-old children from urban and suburban environments.

Introduction Examples

The introduction may conveniently be presented in four basic parts. *The opening comment* is often a broad summarizing statement referring to general interest in the topic:

"The literature of voice disorders consistently indicates the only way to determine the presence or absence of vocal nodules is through a laryngoscopic examination."

(Dice and Shearer, 1973, p. 142)

"It has long been recognized that the introduction of a vent into an otherwise tightly sealed earmold results in a change in the acoustic filter action of the earmold."

(Franks *et al.* 1977, p. 6)

Secondly, some *reference to previous studies* should be made:

"The value of sentence repetition responses in language impaired individuals has been recognized (Berry-Luterman and Bar, 1971; Dukes and Panagos, 1973) and has formed the basis for screening devices (Lee, 1970; Stephens, 1974) and assessment instruments (Carrow, 1974; Spreen and Benton, 1969)."

(Stephens, 1976, p. 493)

"Studies with adults have demonstrated the general influence of syntax on speech perception and production (Greene, 1972), and its peculiar influence on the perception and production of prosodic (Bever, 1970; Goldman-Eisler, 1972) and segmental (Boomer and Laver, 1968; Panagos, 1974b) features."

(Schmauch *et al.*, 1978, p. 315)

Next, it is appropriate to point out how the available information is inadequate, incomplete, scarce, or otherwise in *need of further development*. This statement is to present the reason for conducting the present study, by showing a deficient area which should be filled in by additional results.

"There is clear evidence of reduced intelligibility in dysarthric adults (Tikofsky and Tikofsky, 1964; Tikofsky, Glattke, and Tikofsky, 1966; Tikofsky, 1970), but these studies have not specifically included numbers of subjects with cerebral palsy."

(Platt *et al.*, 1980, p. 29)

"In general, measurement of clinical behavior has been attempted with instruments comprised of relatively few questions which, for the most part, have not been subjected to appropriate item analysis."

(Giolas *et al.*, 1979, p. 169)

At the end of the introduction a clear statement of the *purpose of the study* should be made. The experienced reader of research articles pays particular attention to this part of the introduction because it usually poses the questions which are to be answered later in the results section.

"The purpose of this study, therefore, was to investigate the visual perception of vowels and diphtong phonemes from two horizontal viewing angles, 0° and 90°, in an attempt to answer the following questions:

1. Are diphtongs easier to identify visually than vowels?
2. What differences exist in the visual perception of vowels and diphtongs when observed from horizontal viewing of 0° and 90°?
3. Do orderly, predictable confusions occur among vowel and diphtong phonemes?"

(Wozniak and Jackson, 1979, p. 356)

"The purpose of this study was to provide additional information about pharyngeal wall configuration and displacement and to describe the relationship between these variables and velar displacement."

(Iglesias *et al.*, 1980, p. 430)

Outline of the Introduction

The four points in the preceding section—introductory statement, citation of related studies, shortcomings of previous investigations, and statement of the purpose of the study—may be readily seen in the context of the following introduction:

1. *General introductory statement*

2. *Citation of related studies*

3. *Shortcomings of previous investigations*

"Most articulation tests designed for children use the spontaneous method of response elicitation. However, sometimes the examiner has to ask a child to repeat or imitate a stimulus item, especially when testing preschool children. The problem of whether an imitative method of eliciting responses influences the articulation test results has been studied by several investigators (Seigel *et al.*, 1963; Smith and Ainsworth, 1967; Snow and Milisen, 1954; Templin, 1947; Templin; 1969). These studies have led to differing opinions concerning the effects of imitation on the child's articulatory responses. Of these studies, only one includes preschool children. Templin (1947) tested 100 preschool and kindergarten children (the number of children per age level was not stated). Her results indicated that the differences among the articulation scores were not statistically significant when eliciting responses by the spontaneous and imitative methods. She concluded, "Since neither the spontaneous nor imitative method is superior, the method best adapted to the needs of a specific child can be used."

4. *Statment of the purpose of the study*

To our knowledge no study other than Templin's has been conducted on a population of 4-year-old children. Therefore, it was the purpose of this study to further investigate the effects of spontaneous and imitative methods of response elicitation on articulation test scores for a population of 4-year-old children. Specifically, we sought an answer to the following question: Is there a difference in 4-year-old children's articulation test scores when they are presented two methods of articulation testing—spontaneous and imitative?"
(Kresheck and Socolofsky, 1972, p. 729, by permission of the authors and the *Journal of Speech and Hearing Research*.)

Review of the Literature

In the thesis or dissertation, the literature is reviewed in the section designated as chapter 2. Although references to the literature should also be included as needed in the other chapters, the bulk of the material is presented in one systematically organized section. At the beginning of the chapter, some introductory comments are usually made, which summarize the scope, limitations, and categories to be used in the review.

Particularly in topics where a large amount of literature is available, it is realistic to present only the most relevant citations or to restrict the review to a certain time period or to certain topical areas.

A statement of the scope and limitations might read as:

"The vast amount of literature available on the topic of hearing aids is considerably beyond the intended scope of this study. Therefore the review will be limited to studies dealing only with ear-level aids published during the past ten years."

The categories to be used in the review are often summarized in the introductory comments:

"Articles relating to the general topic of this study are summarized under the headings of Feedback Problems, Amplitude Characteristics, Frequency Characteristics, and Experimental Models."

A few articles which may represent models of the current investigation should be described in all the detail necessary to show the reader everything considered to be important. In some instances, a paragraph or two may be needed for this type of analysis over one article. For the majority of references, however, a single summary statement may encompass a group of three to five related articles.

The compact style of a good literary review is seen in the example which follows. It should be noticed that the review itself is in the form of a flowing narrative, which weaves the references smoothly into the content as the narrative progresses.

"Historically, while speech testing was first used to evaluate speech transmission systems (Egan, 1948), the phonetically balanced word lists (PBs) were soon used to reflect a listener's 'hearing loss for speech' rather than transmission line fidelity (Hirsh, 1947).

Investigations of speech testing methods (Hudgins *et al.*, Pollack *et al.*, 1959) indicated that listener performance was better for known rather than unknown message sets. Oyer and Doudna (1959) observed that response errors decreased with multiple repetition of the CID W-22 lists, suggesting that a closed-response set paradigm be utilized in speech testing. Oyer and Doudna (1959) and Schultz (1964) noticed more errors for vowels than for consonants; they suggested development of a test for vowel discrimination.

House *et al.* (1965) combined the structure of the Fairbanks Rhyme Test (1958) with Pollack's observation that a closed-response set system allows for more reliable test results than an open or quasi-open response set (The Modified Rhyme Test for Consonants (MTR)). Griffiths (1967) produced a further refinement with his minimal-contrast MRT. The House MRT stipulated only that CVC response items be identical for the five possible answers. Griffiths imposes the additional criterian that each response item differ from the test item by a single consonantal feature. The featural contrasts were established on the basis of place and manner of articulation. Ordinary orthographic representation of the word stems had to be abandoned in some cases.

Kreul *et al.* (1968) in turn modified House's MRT in the interests of clinical feasibility. The MRT was partitioned into 6 lists of 50 stimulus items each, the response space was increased to 6 possible answers, and the test was standardized on normal-hearing Ss at 4 S/N ratios. The vowel was constant for all response items."

(Franks and Daniloff, 1973, p. 355, by permission)

METHOD

The section describing the details in which the study was conducted is sometimes tiresome to write and often boring to read, but it is ultimately the most critical part of the research report. Particularly when similar studies yield differing results, the rigor exercised in the methodology may distinguish careful conclusions from hasty observations. The results of any study are only as sound as the method used to obtain them.

The part of the report which is entitled *method* or *procedure* should include a description of the subjects, the apparatus, the manner in which the tests were administered, instructions to subjects, materials used, and sometimes the arrangement or preparation of the data prior to statistical treatment.

1. Subjects

Nearly every research report begins with some description of the subjects used in the study. Depending upon how critical the subjects are to the study, this description may run from as little as one or two sentences to a maximum of several paragraphs. Typically, the considerations of subjects include age, sex, and classification as to type or severity of disorder or normal subjects. Language studies, as mentioned in earlier chapters, usually include about three ages of children, two or three ethnic or regional categories, and several test instruments or linguistic categories.

If normal subjects are used, relatively little description is necessary. In many cases formal testing of speech and hearing is not used, and a subjective evaluation of normality may meet the needs of the study.

"Twenty-five adults, including 20 females and 5 males served as subjects in this study. The subjects ranged in age from 19 to 30 years. None had a history of craniofacial anomalies and all were judged to produce speech normally, including appropriate oral-nasal resonance balances."

(Iglesias *et al.*, 1980, p. 431)

"Subjects for the present investigation were eight adults (five female, three male) ranging in age from 20 to 28 years. None of the subjects had any history of orofacial pathology or functional speech disorder, and each subject reported having normal hearing at the time of testing."

(Weismer and Longstreth, 1980, p. 385)

Where the study is to evaluate special types of sensitive tests, such as hearing tests, the subjects must be selected with somewhat more specific criteria:

One hundred subjects were recruited from an urban public school system. The subjects consisted of 51 males and 49 females, ranging from 7 years, 6 months to 10 years, 6 months. No youngster had failed any previous screening test and none had ever taken the LOT test. Each subject was assumed to be of normal intelligence. None of the youngsters included in the study had hearing thresholds which exceeded 20 dB HL, re ANSI (1969) for the test frequencies 500, 100, 2000, and 4000 Hz."

(Behnke and Lankford, 1976, p. 500, by permission)

Finally, where various categories of clinical disorders or severities are to be compared, each category must be clearly defined.

"Additional language testing placed each patient within a general aphasia syndrome. Two of the five patients were classified as presenting Global aphasia, two were classified as presenting Mixed aphasia, and one was classified as presenting Broca's aphasia."

(Laughlin *et al.*, 1979, p. 312)

2. Instrumentation, materials, and stimuli

This part of the methodology should be described as efficiently as possible, so as to include enough information to allow for replication of the study, but not so much that the description become tedious and belabored with nonessential details. In this section compound sentences are particularly helpful in reducing length and wordiness of the descriptions.

Apparatus

"The carrier signal to the impedance bridge was produced by a Hewlett-Packard Wide Range Oscillator, Model 200 CD. From the impedance bridge (Model E8872A) the signal was picked up by a small crystal type microphone and amplified by a Bruel and Kjaer VTVM. The null was adjusted by using a General Radio Tuned Amplifier, type 1232A. Tape recordings were made on a two channel Magnecord, Model 748-4, and later transferred to graph paper tracings through a Grass Polygraph, Model 5."

(Shearer and Simmons, 1965, p. 205, by permission)

Materials

This classification includes objects or test materials which are used to gather data. This might include descriptions of toys:

"The response set consisted of 14 small objects and body parts of the subject.

The objects included a red truck, blue car, white doll, yellow ring, play wristwatch, three crayons (yellow, black and green), three 2″ × 2″ squares of colored paper (black, red, and green), and three 1″ diameter balls.''

(Panagos and King, 1975, p. 656)

Stimuli

"A set of 24 sentences (see Appendix) was selected for use in the sentence repetition task. Twelve sentences were in a Black English dialect, and 12 were parallel sentences in a Standard English dialect.''

(Stephens, 1976, p. 496)

3. Procedure

The procedure part of the methods section is a simple, matter-of-fact description of everything that happened during the collection of data. Readers who skim through the study are apt to pass over the procedure and to focus more on the abstract and results sections. However, when the study is critically evaluated and being compared with other work the procedure and the design receive the most careful scrutiny. For this reason considerable attention to detail and accuracy must be devoted to this area.

The writing of procedure is not actually difficult, since it is merely the chronical of events carried out by the experimenter. However, the journalistic task is made particularly tedious because of the myriad of fine details which must all be described at the same time. Many of the details can be woven together in compound sentences, which reduce the otherwise choppy nature of the contents. The amount of detail deemed necessary is partly dependent upon the commonality of the techniques used; greater description is required for more unique methods, whereas standardized methods may simply be cited with very little description:

"The measurement criteria outlined by Peterson and Lehiste (1960) were applied to the vowel duration measurements.''

(Adams and Ramig, 1980, p. 460)

Otherwise, the essential criterion is to include enough detail for the study to be duplicated:

"Every session began with a training period in which the subjects first reviewed the phonetic symbols for the 15 vowels. Each subject was then tested on the identification of the items placed at the beginning of each tape and wrote his responses on the back of the answer sheet. Following this, the remainder of the tape containing the 120 stimulus pairs was viewed with dissimilarity ratings being made on a 1–7 scale with 1 being given to pairs which were extremely different. A short rest period was provided after every 25 ratings in order to minimize the fatigue factor.''

(Jackson et al., 1976, p. 800, by permission)

Reliability

The inclusion of reliability of the test measures is not always necessary, particularly when a standardized test is used, on which the reliability is already known. Most standardized audiological procedures, for example, have been evaluated extensively for reliability. However, when a subjective element is implied in the measure, the test should be repeated in order to verify the constancy of the data. The concept of reliability and the methods involved are discussed in an earlier section entitled Research Concepts and Terminology.

In most instance, procedures used to establish reliability appear in two forms. The first is judges' reliability. This can consist both of interjudge reliability, which means the comparison of one judge's evaluative results with those of another judge, or in intrajudge reliability, which means the comparison of a judge's scores with those of his later scores on the same test. This type of reliability is needed in situations where the data must be derived in the form of clinical judgments on performance or observations of characteristics. These might include relative hoarseness, clinical progress, aesthetic effect, or other entities which do not ordinarily appear as numerical information. Common reliability techniques in these instances are correlations between scores, and percentage of agreement.

The second widely used area of reliability is where numerical measures depend upon the degree of precision which might vary from one individual to the next. A common example is in the measures of X-ray pictures for the study of speech movements or velar insufficiency in cleft palate cases. Occasionally, similarly difficult measures are conducted on strip chart recordings or spectrographs. In this type of reliability the *standard error of the mean* is frequently used. For instance, the standard error in X-ray measures is usually in the order of .5 millimeters, which means that when two individuals measure the same picture their measurements agree within one-half millimeter.

"Interjudge reliability then was caluclated by comparing the decisions from the taped responses of each of the five clinicians with those of the examiner on initial testing. Interjudge reliability averaged across the five clinicians, the five children, and all sounds was 93.9% on the DTA and 92.6% on the AAAPS."

(Schissel and James, 1979, p. 366)

"Mean agreements between the experimenter and the first observer were 90 and 87% for sound production tasks and talking tasks, respectively. Agreements of 88 and 85% were obtained between the experimenter and the second observer for the two measures."

(Ruscello and Shelton, 1979, p. 506)

"Correlation coefficients (Huntsberger and Leaverton, 1970) of agreement between observers were calculated for the events with high positive correlation coefficients ranging from +0.96 to +1.00. The results suggest a very high degree of reliability between observers in judging the performances of the subject."

(Cottrel *et al.*, 1980, p. 94)

4. Data Arrangement

The section on data arrangement is an optional part of the methods category of the report. In most cases there are no special techniques in arranging the data since it is already self-evident in the procedure. In audiology, nothing needs to be said about the clinical results if they are already in the form of hearing thresholds or discrimination scores. In speech pathology or language, the standardized tests and measures are equally evident. However, if some unique types of data are used or if the arrangement is a bit more complicated, an extra short paragraph may be necessary. Particularly in a thesis or dissertation, where printing space is not the problem it becomes in published articles, some comment on data arrangement is more likely to be added at the end of the Methods chapter.

Sometimes the data arrangement in the form of the type of experimental design is added for clarity, to prepare the reader for the results chapter. In other examples, some relatively novel measurements require additional explanation in order to make the data replicable to other researchers.

Statistical Analysis

The inclusion of statistical analysis is another optional aspect of the Methods section. Where the results are based upon rather routine and uncomplicated treatments, such as t-tests or simple analyses of variance, the description is hardly necessary. A more common approach is to set forth the statistical procedures in the opening pargraph of the Results. However, where the data are to be divided into some special patterns prior to statistical analysis, such arrangements are often included in the last paragraph of the Methods.

"The independent variables were (1) urban groups: City A-black, City B-black, City A-white, City B-white, City A-Spanish-speaking; (2) sex; (3) feature; and (4) dialectal form of the feature. Variables 3 and 4 were repeated measures factors. The dependent variable was success in repeating the sentences and was measured, as noted previously, using three scoring procedures, necessitating three analyses of variance."

(Stephens, 1976, p. 498)

RESULTS

The results chapter is read more than any other part of the written report, except the abstract. It is the systematic presentation of each part of the research questions which have been raised, along with a definitive answer to each item. Additional descriptions of special data arrangements, computer programs, or innovative statistical procedures may also be included as deemed helpful to the understanding of the study.

In a well-organized presentation, the outline for the Results is already implied in the last paragraph of the *Introduction*, particularly if the research questions have been spelled out in a numerical outline. The results are then taken up one at a time in their original order. Tentatively, a paragraph should be visualized for each part of the results. Each result should state the question to be answered, the statistic used, the numerical result, and the conclusion drawn from the result.

The most common opening statement for the results section is to direct the reader's attention to a chart, table, graph, or other summary of the data:

"Table 1 shows the comprehension performance of the normal and deviant-speaking children on the high and low-intelligibility sentences. With the exception of the deviant-speaking subject's tendency to respond more frequently to their own utterances, the performances of the group were similar on both types of sentences."

(Panagos and King, 1975, p. 658)

At other times, it may seem most appropriate to begin with a reference to the type of statistic or the experimental design employed in establishing the results:

"Total scores for the receptive section and expressive section initially were analyzed within a two-way analysis of variance for the effects of sex and age of children. Boys and girls performed similarly on the receptive ($F = 1.56$; $df = 1,880$; NS) and expressive ($F = 1.72$; $df = 1,880$; NS) portions of the NSST."

(Ratusnik et al, 1980, p. 202)

If a general opening statement is unnecessary, the first sentence should be the first part of the results, in the order of the questions raised.

"An examination of impedance results revealed that 52% (41) of the 79 children screened failed tympanometry."

(Bruns et al., 1979, p. 56)

A more direct approach to the results is to lead off in the opening statement with what might be termed the "punch line" to the study, i.e., the most important part of the results:

"First, the hypothesis that language proficiency as measured by MLU, is correlated with accuracy of articulation was not supported for either language-delayed or for normal-speaking children."

(Bond and Wilson, 1980, p. 155)

Speculation and far reaching implications gleaned from the data should be included in the discussion rather than in the results chapter, but brief comments which give the reader the importance of each group of analyses should be included for each aspect of the result.

Although bold and uncompromising statements about results should be made with caution, research writing should not be so completely qualified as to present the reader with vague uncertainties. The acceptable phraseology is usually "results indicate . . . ," or "results suggest . . . ." More carefully reserved statements would be, "results seem to indicate . . . ," or "results would suggest . . . ."

Strictly speaking, the results section need not have a designated ending; most do not. This part of the report simply concludes in most instances with the last point to be made in the series of data analyses. Any comments which would help to tie the results together or to point out their implications are typically left for the Discussion section at the end of the report. In a few instances, however, the Results section is concluded in a more deliberate manner, helping the reader to picture the main points a bit more clearly:

"In summary, a DAF effect on nonfluencies was not found for the adults. The children did respond to the delays with an increase in nonfluencies, but for the most part, the various delay intervals were equally disturbing."

(Siegel et al., 1980, p. 810)

An alternative ending is to prepare the reader for the Discussion section, which is to follow:

"These data raise the question of the degree to which preference judgments of hearing-aid processed speech are transitive when characteristics other than low-cutoff frequency vary concurrently, that is, when actual hearing aids are used.''

(Punch and Beck, 1980, p. 333)

DISCUSSION

The last section of the written report is typically designated as the Discussion. This part of the report, however, is not quite as standard as are the other sections or chapters. The last section may, for example, be designated as Clinical Implications, Discussion and Conclusions, Summary, or the discussion aspect of the report is simply omitted.

The discussion, however, serves a very useful purpose in the report, because a reader having particular interest in that area usually is interested, not only in the results, per se, but also what the researcher's opinion is about the study in general and the place it seems to have in the total picture of the discipline. It is here that the author offers suggestions for therapy, ideas for future research, or enters into some current controversy in opposition or in support of other research works. Basically, it intends to answer the question, "What does it all mean?"

The opening comment of the Discussion is appropriately a summary of the main thrust of the study. Quite commonly, this statement also refers to similar results from parallel studies:

"These results lend support to the hypothesis that syntax influences the accuracy of consonant production in language-disordered children. Simply stated, a language-disordered child is more likely to misarticulate a target consonant in a sentence context than in an isolated noun phrase context."

(Schmauch *et al.*, 1978, p. 320)

"The most obvious finding of this study is the reconfirmation of the fact that most obvious black children's oral language production is presently stronger in black English than in Standard English. This result was demonstrated earlier for elementary school children in Washington, D.C., (Baratz, 1969), and for 5-year-olds in Baltimore (Osser et al, 1969). Also, this study presents additional evidence of linguistic interference when black children attempt to use Standard English forms."

(Stephens, 1976, p. 503)

The body of the discussion may bring out supplementary aspects of the study, such as alternate ways to interpret the results, reservations or cautions about the conclusions, or special strengths or effectiveness of the methods used.

Interpretation:

"A reasonable explanation of our data is that subjects perceived their voices as increasing in nasality under low-pass filtering and attempted to compensate by decreasing nasalization. There is evidence that speakers sometimes do make compensatory changes in speech when their feedback is modified."

(Garber and Moller, 1979, p. 329)

Reservations and Cautions:

"Interpretation of the results must be tempered by the recognition that the findings have not been replicated. However, the position shared by several theories indicating stuttering is acquired and maintained by neurological cues which, after association with punishment, elicit negative emotionality may be too simplistic."

(Reed and Lingwell, 1980, p. 343)

Effectiveness of the Method:

"Finally, the time-point analysis technique used in this study proved to be an effective objective procedure for scoring and analyzing the neonate's middle components of the AER. Once the time-points were calculated, all of the AER scoring and analysis was accomplished by machine, additing objectivity while simultaneously reducing analysis time."

(Wolf and Goldstein, 1980, p. 1980)

The Discussion most often ends with a statement regarding the questions which are still unanswered, or problems which are still unresolved, conveying a message to the reader that the study has brought us further in our understanding of the topic, but more conclusions are still to be sought.

"As we did not make perceptual judgments of subjects' nasality productions, it is difficult to determine whether these changes in nasalization were clinically significant. Further investigation is necessary before we can determine whether filtering may be useful clinically as a method of reducing nasality."

(Garber and Moller, 1979, p. 330)

"Additional data from other laboratories will be required to establish further the validity of these findings. Furthermore, data must be accumulated to verify the accuracy of the other available types of hearing test equipment."

(Townsend, 1980, p. 334)

Studies, however, which deal with more immediate, rather than theoretical questions are inclined to end the discussion with a conclusive statement or recommendation.

"It was concluded on the basis of the test results, child observation, and parent reaction that an educative approach to vocal hygiene benefitted children exhibiting hoarse voices. This program would be of benefit to school speech-language pathologists who deal with large number of children exhibiting hoarseness."

(Cook et al., 1979, p. 24)

ABSTRACT

Most journals and convention programs require that submitted manuscripts be accompanied by an abstract of the written work. An abstract is also required as part of the thesis or dissertation. As a rule the maximum length of the abstract is precisely specified, such as "do not exceed 75 words" for ASHA Convention abstracts, or "an abstract not to exceed 200 words" for the *Journal of Speech and Hearing Disorders* and the *Journal of Speech and Hearing Research*. Longer abstracts may run as long as a full page or more. Although the criteria which distinguish abstracts from summaries are not well defined, it is found that summaries are generally longer than abstracts and normally appear at the end of the report, whereas abstracts are nearly always at the beginning.

The primary purpose of the abstract is to give the reader enough information to decide whether he or she should read (or hear, in the case of a convention paper) the full length report. With this purpose in mind, the most efficient abstract should be short enough to be read almost at a glance. In complicated studies this extreme level of condensation may not always be realistic or practical. From the standpoint of both time and expense, however, it is well to consider the abstract in its role as part of our growing library reference retrieval systems. Unnecessarily long wording in the abstracts serves only to reduce the efficiency of these types of reference media.

When brevity is the prime consideration for the abstract, it can become a factor of extreme frustration for the inexperienced writer, who can see no way to throw out any of the "critical details" of the study in order to fall within the maximum number of words allowed. The critical details, no matter how carefully developed, belong in the full report—not in the abstract. When the length of the abstract comes close to fitting the requirements a few words can sometimes be saved here and there by using a longer compound sentence rather than several short ones. For example, a compound sentence such as,

"Subjects were evaluated by pure tone thresholds for 500 through 2000 Hz, SRTs and discrimination scores, to establish hearing adequacy and type of hearing loss."

requires fewer words than the individual shorter sentences,

"Subjects were evaluated by pure tone thresholds, SRTs, and discrimination scores. Pure tones were 500 through 2000 Hz. The tests were used to establish hearing adequacy and type of hearing loss."

The briefest abstract of any research study can be stated adequately in three sentences. The *first* sentence should state the basic concept of the study. The *second* sentence describes the method used in obtaining the results, and the *third* sentence contains the results and/or the implications of the study.

Concept: "This study dealt with the influence of two methods of assessing articulation upon the articulation scores of 45 four-year-old children.

Method: The children were tested by both an imitative and spontaneous method of articulatory assessment on each of 87 words taken from the Templin-Darley Tests of Articulation.

Results: The results indicated a significant difference between the two methods of stimulus presentation in the children's total articulation scores."

(Kresheck and Socolofsky, 1972, p. 729)

The same basic outline is illustrated again in a somewhat shorter example:

Concept: "A system for the study of phonation by high-speed photography is described. The data were extracted from the film by tracing

Method: the glottal areas and waveform amplitudes with a pantograph. The temperature rise produced by the intense illumination re-

Results: quired for the photography was found to be moderate and safe."

(Soron, 1967, p. 768)

THE PROSPECTUS

It is customary for the student embarking upon a thesis or dissertation to submit an outline of his or her proposed undertaking for evaluation by a faculty committee. This may vary from a rough narrative sketch or simple outline to as much as the first three completed chapters for the finished study. An initial summary, or prospectus, however, is not limited to graduate student research projects, but is also typically required in grant proposals or other endeavors in which permission, time, or other support is requested for research purposes. This simplest and most efficient form of the prospectus is a miniature or perhaps microscopic version of the thesis/dissertation.

Particularly in the case of the dissertation, the prospectus is sometimes considered to be the completed first draft of the Introduction, Review of Literature, and Method sections of the written work. When this approach is used, the initial brief outline is called the *pre-prospectus*, which is still a part of the original formative planning for the intended project. Regardless of length, however, it is essential that the prospectus will enable the reader to grasp the significance of the study as well as the feasibility of completing the study in the allotted amount of time using the facilities available. The most helpful form for the prospectus consists of about five pages, with each page summarizing what is to be included in one chapter of the thesis. The outline for the five chapters of a typical thesis are outlined earlier in this section of the text, and may be used as a guide for writing the prospectus.

Since there is usually no abstract to accompany the prospectus, the *Introductory* page should give the reader all he needs to know about the intended project, and what its results might contribute. The abbreviated *Review of the Literature* should refer particularly to any study or group of studies which are most parallel to the intended project, or to a study which might serve as a model for the present investigation. If related literature is particularly scarce this point should be explained in the prospectus since it represents a consideration to be discussed in the planning sessions.

The *Method* section should be given special attention since this is the section which must serve as the blueprint for conducting the study. In particular, it should specify the subjects to be used and the availability of any apparatus or facilities required. It should also demonstrate clearly that the procedure and measures will yield the type of data needed to answer fully the questions contained in the hypothesis. Particularly when the research topic is unique, having little directly related suportive material from the literature, a small pilot study employing from one to five subjects is desirable for presentation in the prospectus.

The *Results* and *Discussion* are not always included in the prospectus on the assumption that the data must first be collected before these sections could be visualized. However, some thought should be devoted to these two areas which raise some important questions to be resolved before the project is underway. In the results section, the planned statistic should be outlined in advance, along with any proposed tables and graphs. Results of the pilot study might also be included in this section. The Discussion, if included, is the section which shows how the results might relate with those from other studies, and points out some of the tentative implicatiaons which could be made. Since most research serves to open rather than to close the door on an area of discovery, the implications should be viewed as part of a continuum rather than the final conclusion.

The Prospectus Meeting

A prospectus meeting is held for the purpose of reviewing the research proposal and evaluating its strengths, weaknesses, feasibility, and probable contribution. Although some criticism may be offered, the general tone of the meeting is positive and geared toward helpful suggestions from the faculty committee. Usually the committee consists of the thesis/dissertation advisor and two or more additional faculty members chosen by the student. For the doctoral dissertation, the committee customarily has another member invited from outside the student's academic department, although he does not necessarily participate in the planning stages of the study and in fact may not appear until the oral defense of the completed dissertation. Since the advisor is usually very well versed in the research topic to be investigated, the other members of the committee might be chosen because they view the topic from different perspectives or can serve as valuable consultants in statistics, instrumentation, or other aspects of the investigation. The primary responsibility of the committee during the prospectus meeting is to evaluate and approve the student's research proposal, usually with suggestions to make the design a bit tighter or to make the endeavor generally more realistic within the scope of the student's time and resources. Approval of the prospectus is based on the assumption that the student will generally incorporate the committee's suggestions and that the committee will be generally inclined to accept the thesis or dissertation if it is carried out according to the approved plan. Ideally, then, the prospectus meeting should conclude in a spirit of mutual agreement, and the tacit acceptance of mutual responsibility.

TITLE OF THE STUDY

Typically, the title is added to the study after it is written in its entirety. Titles are not particularly difficult to write, and in comparison with the rest of the written work they are perhaps even considered unimportant. However, as the volume of information increases and computerized bibliographies become more commonplace the length and content of titles must be evaluated more carefully. Anyone who has assembled an extensive bibliography shares an appreciation of short, efficiently worded titles.

It is not necessary to include all of the variables and all of the concepts of the study into the title, although it is generally accepted that the titles of theses and dissertations may be more elaborately phrased than those of published articles or convention papers. A certain amount of preamble and flowery prose is tolerated in the titles of graduate student research and it is not unusual to find phraseology such as "A Preliminary Investigation and Factor Analysis of Selected Variables Which Could Influence the Diminution or Elimination of Secondary Symptoms in Stuttering Behavior." This elaborate literary style is a holdover from a previous age, and although it conveys an admirable scholarly tone, it does not train the student for the efficient terminology needed in the computer age.

Nearly all studies are based mainly upon two or three basic concepts, which should be conveyed in the title. Supplemetary concepts, explanatory phrases, and extra adjectives may make a more comprehensive title, but any words which do not contribute critical information should probably be omitted. A few examples of efficient titles are:

"Speech Performance, Dysphasia, and Oral Reflexes in Cerebral Palsy."

(Love et al., 1980)

"Hearing Levels Among Elderly Nursing Home Residents"

(Schow and Nerbonne, 1980)

"Two-Tone Foreward Masking Patterns and Tinnitus"

(Penner, 1980)

"Delayed Auditory Feedback with Children"

(Siegel *et al.*, 1980)

It should be noted that verbs, extra adjectives, and connecting words are implied rather than stated in these examples, but the basic concepts of the studies are included.

ACKNOWLEDGMENT PAGE OF THE THESIS OR DISSERTATION

The acknowledgment page near the front of the graduate student research report is somewhat analogous to the preface in a book. Whereas a preface shares with the reader the reasons and circumstances for writing the book, and includes those who aided in information and editing, the thesis/dissertation acknowledgment is a relatively standardized mention of the student's research committee.

Although the protocol is not rigid, it is customary to mention first the faculty advisor of the study, and then to mention the other members of the committee as a group. Depending upon the type and amount of assistance provided, the faculty advisor should be thanked for his/her time, guidance, patience, or direction given to the study. This is usually phrased as "I would like to thank" or "The author wishes to express his appreciation."

If the committee members each made a separate type of contribution a more individual style for acknowledgment might be in order: "I would like to thank Dr. David Williams for his careful editing of the manuscript, Dr. John Franks for his computer assistance, and Dr. Earl Seaver for his help with the measurment techniques."

In addition to acknowledging the faculty committee members for their time and services, the student may also wish to express appreciation to a spouse, parents, or other family members who made some special contribution or supportive effort toward the successful completion of the study. Finally, there may have been other supportive individuals, without whose help the study may not have been completed. This individual may have supplied subjects, case files, or access to the use of special facilities. Overall, the acknowledgments should be stated simply, without additional narrative or detail, typically amounting to a page or a page and a half.

In published research, an acknowledgment section is considered optional, except when the study was sponsored by a grant or if a significant part of the study, such as subjects, test material, or data files were made available by some agency or individual. While it is not necessary to mention the routine assistance and advice which one might receive from colleagues while conducting the study and preparing the manuscript, the majority of current articles do contain some type of acknowledgment, varying from one brief sentence to as much as a paragraph of 100 words or more.

BIBLIOGRAPHIC REFERENCE

Few journals use exactly the same reference style, since each adopts a method which seems to suite its own needs. Generally speaking, journals dealing with clinical and experimental topics tend to use simpler reference styles and fewer footnotes than do those of a more literary nature.

Unfortunately, some of the reference styles used in theses, dissertations, and term papers are patterned upon traditional forms which are never used in actual publication, and the student would seem to be better prepared for his/her career by employing the reference styles from the journals in his field.

The examples which follow are taken from the *Journal of Speech and Hearing Research*, the *Journal of Speech and Hearing Disorders*, and *Language, Speech, and Hearing Services in Schools*, which use identical styles. It is interesting to note that as late as 1968 it was accepted practice to use the first initial for male authors, while female authors were referenced with their name spelled out in full.

Journal Articles

Single author:
> Panagos, J., Persistence of the open syllable reinterpreted as a symptom of language disorders. *J. Speech Hearing Dis.*, 39, 23–31 (1974).

Two authors:
> Miller, G., and Nicely, P., An analysis of perceptual confusions among some English consonants. *J. Acoust. Soc. Amer.*, 27, 338–352 (1955).

More than two authors:
> Binnie, C., Montgomery, A., and Jackson, P., Auditory and visual contributions to the perception of consonants. *J. Speech Hearing Res.*, 17, 619–630 (1974).

Journal supplement:
> Sonesson, B., On the anatomy and vibratory pattern of the human vocal folds. *Acta Otolaryng.*, suppl. 156, 7–80, (1960).

Technical Reports

Lindqvist, J., A descriptive model of laryngeal articulation in speech. *Quart. Prog. Stat. Rep.* Speech Transmission Laboratory, Stockholm, 2–3/1972, 1–9 (1972).

Books

Standard reference:
> Siegel, S., *Nonparametric Statistics for the Behavioral Sciences.* New York: McGraw-Hill (1956).

Specific edition:
> Van Riper, C., *Speech Correction: Principles and Methods.* (6th ed.) Englewood Cliffs, N.J.: Prentice-Hall (1978).

Specific chapter:
> Katz, J., The staggered spondaic word test. In R. Keith (Ed.), *Central Auditory Dysfunction.* New York: Grune and Stratton (1977).

Doctoral Dissertation

Kuehn, D., A cinefluorographic investigation of articulatory velocities. Doctoral dissertation, Univ. of Iowa (1973).

Master's Thesis

Carson, P., A comparison of learning by deaf children through seven conditions of communication. Master's Thesis, Univ. of Kansas (1974).

Unpublished Manuscript

Chatelantat, G., and Schoggen, M., An observation system of assessment of spontaneous infant behavior. Unpublished manuscript, George Peabody College (1975).

Convention Paper

Cerf, A., and Prins, D., Stutterers' ear preference for dichotic syllables. Paper presented to the American Speech-Language-Hearing Association Convention, Las Vegas (1974).

Abstract

Allred, P., McCandless, G., and Weaver, R., Tympanometry and the emergence of the acoustic reflex in neonates. (abstract) *Asha*, 16, 564 (1974).

Test Materials

Goldman, R., Fristoe, M., and Woodcock, R., *Goldman-Fristoe-Woodcock Auditory Skills Test Battery.* Circle Pines, Minnesota: American Guidance Service (1976).

Secondary Reference Source

(This form may be used when the original source is not available, but has been cited by another author.)

Bruno, C., cited by Block, P., Neuro-psychiatric aspects of spastic dysphonia. *Folia Phoniatrica*, 17, 301–364 (1965).

Several References by the Same Author and Same Year

In the text a letter is added to the author's name and year, as in reference to Fromkin (1966a).

Fromkin, V., Neuromuscular specification of linguistic units. *Lang. Speech*, 9, 170–199 (1966a).

Fromkin, V., Some requirements for a model of performance. *UCLA Working Papers in Phonetics*, No. 4, 19–39 (1966b).

Personal Communication

(This reference may be included in the body of the text with no bibliographic reference at the end of the article.) The following is from Webster and Lubker (1968, p. 765):

"Procedures are being developed to facilitate carryover of fluent speech patterns into situations outside the laboratory (Goldiamond, personal communication, 1967)."

Appendices

Appendix A

Answers to Exercises

1. #1. t-test for Independent Groups
   #2. Treatments-by-Subjects AOV
   #3. Friedman's Test
   #4. Cochran's Q Test
   #5. Proportions Test
   #6. One-way AOV
   #7. Sign Test
   #8. Mann-Whitney U
   #9. Treatments-by-Groups
   #10. Wilcoxon Matched Pairs T
   #11. Pearson r
   #12. t-test for Related Measures
   #13. Spearman Rho
2. $t = 5.01$; $df = 12$
3. $U = 5$; $p = <.02$
4. $P1 = .9$, $P2 = .5$; $z = .14$
5. $t = 29.16$; $df = 6$
6. $T = 3$, $N = 8$, $p = <.05$
7. $z = 2.33$
8. $z = /.58$
9. $F = 31.90$ $df = 2, 12$
10. $H = 12.50$; $df = 2$
11. $F = 19.74$; $df = 2, 8$
12. $X^2 = 11.64$; $df = 3$
13. $Q = 3.92$
14. F (Groups) $= 1.10$; F (Treatments) $= 467.11$; F (Interaction) $= 9.33$
15. F (factor A) :eq 7.53; F (factor B) $= 53.89$; F (Interaction) $= 1.59$
16. $q = 3.95$, SE $= .45$, Critical Difference $= 1.55$
17. SE $= .63$, F factor $= 6.23$, Critical Values $= 3.93$
18. SE $= .45$; 9 value for 3 ranks $= 3.95$, for 2 ranks $= 3.20$; Critical Differences $= 1.44$ and 1.78
19. $\sum X = 104$, $\sum X^2 = 874$, $\sum Y = 113$, $\sum Y^2 = 963$, $r = .96$
20. $\sum D^2 = 14$; rho $= .95$
21. $X^2 = .104$

Appendix B

Sample Format: Doctoral Dissertation

A CINEFLUOROGRAPHIC AND ELECTROMYOGRAPHIC

INVESTIGATION OF VELAR POSITIONING

IN ALL ORAL SPEECH

by

Earl J. Seaver III

A thesis submitted in partial fulfillment of the
requirements for the degree of Doctor of
Philosophy in Speech Pathology and
Audiology in the Graduate College of
The University of Iowa

December, 1978

Thesis Supervisors: Professor Hughlett L. Morris
                        Adjunct Assistant Professor
                        David P. Kuehn

TABLE OF CONTENTS

CHAPTER   Page

LIST OF TABLES

LIST OF FIGURES

Appendix C

Sample Format: Master's Thesis

ABSTRACT

Name: Keely Jade Gilmore   Department: Communication
                                              Disorders

Title: The Effects of Speech-Frequency Masking on
         Selected Vocal Characteristics of Stutterers
         and Nonstutterers

Major: Speech Pathology   Degree: Master of Arts

Approved by: Date:

_____   _____

NORTHERN ILLINOIS UNIVERSITY

NORTHERN ILLINOIS UNIVERSITY

THE EFFECTS OF SPEECH-FREQUENCY MASKING

ON SELECTED VOCAL CHARACTERISTICS OF

STUTTERERS AND NONSTUTTERERS

A THESIS SUBMITTED TO THE GRADUATE SCHOOL

IN PARTIAL FULFILLMENT OF THE REQUIREMENTS

FOR THE DEGREE

MASTER OF ARTS

DEPARTMENT OF COMMUNICATION DISORDERS

BY

KEELY JADE GILMORE

DEKALB, ILLINOIS
JANUARY 1981

Certification: In accordance with departmental and
Graduate School policies, this thesis
is accepted in partial fulfillment of
degree requirements.

_____
Thesis Director

_____
Date

To my two Best Friends

Shirley and Irwin

TABLE OF CONTENTS

LIST OF TABLES

LIST OF FIGURES

LIST OF APPENDIXES

APPENDIX

Appendix D

Table of Square Roots

n	$\sqrt{n}$	n	$\sqrt{n}$	n	$\sqrt{n}$	n	$\sqrt{n}$
1	1.000 00	58	7.615 77	115	10.72381	172	13.11488
2	1.414 21	59	7.618 15	116	10.77033	173	13.15295
3	1.732 05	60	7.745 97	117	10.81665	174	13.19091
4	2.000 00	61	7.810 25	118	10.86278	175	13.22876
5	2.236 07	62	7.874 01	119	10.90871	176	13.26650
6	2449 49	63	7.937 25	120	10.95445	177	13.30413
7	2.645 75	64	8.000 00	121	11.00000	178	13.34166
8	2.828 43	65	8.062 26	122	11.04536	179	13.37909
9	3.000 00	66	8.124 04	123	11.09054	180	13.41641
10	3.162 28	67	8.185 35	124	11.13553	181	13.45362
11	3.316 63	68	8.246 21	125	11.18034	182	13.49074
12	3.464 10	69	8.306 62	126	11.22497	183	13.52775
13	3.605 55	70	8.366 60	127	11.26943	184	13.56466
14	3.741 66	71	8.426 15	128	11.31371	185	13.60147
15	3.872 98	72	8.485 28	129	11.35782	186	13.63818
16	4.000 00	73	8.544 00	130	11.40175	187	13.67479
17	4.123 11	74	8.602 33	131	11.44552	188	13.71131
18	4.242 64	75	8.660 25	132	11.48913	189	13.74773
19	4.358 90	76	8.717 80	133	11.53256	190	13.78405
20	4.472 14	77	8.774 96	134	11.57584	191	13.82027
21	4.582 58	78	8.831 76	135	11.61895	192	13.85641
22	4.690 42	79	8.888 19	136	11.66190	193	13.89244
23	4.795 83	80	8.944 27	137	11.70470	194	13.92839
24	4.898 98	81	9.000 00	138	11.74734	195	13.96424
25	5.000 00	82	9.055 39	139	11.78983	196	14.00000
26	5.099 02	83	9.110 43	140	11.83216	197	14.03567
27	5.196 15	84	9.165 15	141	11.87434	198	14.07125
28	5.291 50	85	9.219 54	142	11.91638	199	14.10674
29	5.385 17	86	9.273 62	143	11.95826	200	14.14214
30	5.477 23	87	9.327 38	144	12.00000	201	14.17745
31	5.567 76	88	9.380 83	145	12.04159	202	14.21267
32	5.656 85	89	9.433 98	146	12.08305	203	14.24781
33	5.744 56	90	9.486 83	147	12.12436	204	14.28286
34	5.830 95	91	9.539 39	148	12.16553	205	14.31782
35	5.916 08	92	9.591 66	149	12.20656	206	14.35270
36	6.000 00	93	9.643 65	150	12.24745	207	14.38749
37	6.082 76	94	9.695 36	151	12.28821	208	14.42221
38	6.164 41	95	9.746 79	152	12.32883	209	14.45683
39	6.245 00	96	9.797 96	153	12.36932	210	14.49138
40	6.324 56	97	9.848 86	154	12.40967	211	14.52584
41	6.403 12	98	9.899 50	155	12.44990	212	14.56022
42	6.480 74	99	9.949 87	156	12.49000	213	14.59452
43	6.557 44	100	10.00000	157	12.52996	214	14.62874
44	6.633 25	101	10.04998	158	12.56981	215	14.66288
45	6.708 20	102	10.09950	159	12.60952	216	14.69694
46	6.782 33	103	10.14889	160	12.64911	217	14.73092
47	6.855 66	104	10.19804	161	12.68858	218	14.76482
48	6.928 20	105	10.24695	162	12.72792	219	14.79865
49	7.000 00	106	10.29563	163	12.76715	220	14.83240
50	7.071 07	107	10.34408	164	12.80625	221	14.86607
51	7.141 43	108	10.39230	165	12.84523	222	14.89966
52	7.211 10	109	10.44031	166	12.88410	223	14.93318
53	7.280 11	110	10.48809	167	12.92285	224	14.96663
54	7.348 47	111	10.53565	168	12.96148	225	15.00000
55	7.416 20	112	10.58301	169	13.00000	226	15.03330
56	7.483 32	113	10.63015	170	13.03840	227	15.06652
57	7.549 83	114	10.67708	171	13.07670	228	15.09967

Appendix D—continued

n	$\sqrt{n}$	n	$\sqrt{n}$	n	$\sqrt{n}$	n	$\sqrt{n}$
229	15.13275	286	16.91153	343	18.52026	400	20.00000
230	15.16575	287	16.94107	344	18.54724	401	20.02498
231	15.19868	288	16.97056	345	18.57418	402	20.04994
232	15.23155	289	17.00000	346	18.60108	403	20.07486
233	15.26434	290	17.02939	347	18.62794	404	20.09975
234	15.29706	291	17.05872	348	18.65476	405	20.12461
235	15.32971	292	17.08801	349	18.68154	406	20.14944
236	15.36229	293	17.11724	350	18.70829	407	20.17424
237	15.39480	294	17.14643	351	18.73499	408	20.19901
238	15.42725	295	17.17556	352	18.76166	409	20.22375
239	15.45962	296	17.20465	353	18.78829	410	20.24864
240	15.49193	297	17.23369	354	18.81489	411	20.27313
241	15.52417	298	17.26268	355	18.84144	412	20.29778
242	15.55635	299	17.29162	356	18.86796	413	20.32240
243	15.58846	300	17.32051	357	18.89444	414	20.34699
244	15.62050	301	17.34935	358	18.92089	415	20.37155
245	15.65248	302	17.37815	359	18.94730	416	20.39608
246	15.68439	303	17.40690	360	18.97367	417	20.42058
247	15.71623	304	17.43560	361	19.00000	418	20.44505
248	15.74902	305	17.46425	362	19.02630	419	20.46949
249	15.77973	306	17.49286	363	19.05256	420	20.49390
250	15.81139	307	17.52142	364	19.07878	421	20.51828
251	15.84298	308	17.54993	365	19.10497	422	20.54264
252	15.87451	309	17.57840	366	19.13113	423	20.56696
253	15.90597	310	17.60682	367	19.15724	424	20.59126
254	15.93738	311	17.63519	368	19.18333	425	20.61553
255	15.96872	312	17.66352	369	19.20937	426	20.63977
256	16.00000	313	17.69181	370	19.23538	427	20.66398
257	16.03122	314	17.72005	371	19.26136	428	20.68816
258	16.06238	315	17.74824	372	19.28730	429	20.71232
259	16.09348	316	17.77639	373	19.31321	430	20.73644
260	16.12452	317	17.80449	374	19.33908	431	20.75054
261	16.15549	318	17.83255	375	19.36492	432	20.78461
262	16.18641	319	17.86057	376	19.39072	433	20.80865
263	16.21727	320	17.88854	377	19.41649	434	20.83267
264	16.24808	321	17.91647	378	19.44222	435	20.85665
265	16.27882	322	17.84436	379	19.46792	436	20.88061
266	16.30951	323	17.97220	380	19.49359	437	20.90454
267	16.34013	324	18.00000	381	19.51922	438	20.92845
268	16.37071	325	18.02776	382	19.54482	439	20.95233
269	16.40122	326	18.05547	383	19.57039	440	20.97618
270	16.43168	327	18.08314	384	19.59592	441	21.00000
271	16.46208	328	18.11077	385	19.63142	442	21.02380
272	16.49242	329	18.13836	386	19.64688	443	21.04757
273	16.52271	330	18.16590	387	19.67232	444	21.07131
274	16.55295	331	18.18341	388	19.69772	445	21.09502
275	16.58312	332	18.22087	389	19.72308	446	21.11871
276	16.61235	333	18.24829	390	19.74842	447	21.14237
277	16.64332	334	18.27567	391	19.77372	448	21.16601
278	16.67333	335	18.30301	392	19.79899	449	21.18962
279	16.70329	336	18.33030	393	19.82423	450	21.21320
280	16.73320	337	18.35756	394	19.84943	451	21.23676
281	16.76305	338	18.38478	395	19.87461	452	21.26029
282	16.79286	339	18.41195	396	19.89975	453	21.28380
283	16.82260	340	18.43909	397	19.92486	454	21.30728
284	16.85230	341	18.46619	398	19.94994	455	21.33073
285	16.88194	342	18.49324	399	19.97498	456	21.35416

Appendix D—continued

n	$\sqrt{n}$	n	$\sqrt{n}$	n	$\sqrt{n}$	n	$\sqrt{n}$
457	21.37756	514	22.67157	571	23.89561	628	25.05993
458	21.40093	515	22.69361	572	23.91652	629	25.07987
459	21.42429	516	22.71563	573	23.93742	630	25.09980
460	21.44761	517	22.73763	574	23.95830	631	25.11971
461	21.47091	518	22.75961	575	23.97916	632	25.13961
462	21.49419	519	22.78157	576	24.00000	633	25.15949
463	21.51743	520	22.80351	577	24.02082	634	25.17936
464	21.54066	521	22.82542	578	24.04163	635	25.19921
465	21.56386	522	22.84732	579	24.06242	636	25.21904
466	21.58703	523	22.86919	580	24.08319	637	25.23886
467	21.61018	524	22.89105	581	24.10394	638	25.25866
468	21.63331	525	22.91288	582	24.12468	639	25.27845
469	21.65641	526	22.93469	583	24.14539	640	25.29822
470	21.67948	527	22.95648	584	24.16609	641	25.31798
471	21.70253	528	22.97825	585	24.18677	642	25.33772
472	21.72556	529	23.00000	586	24.20744	643	25.35744
473	21.74856	530	23.02173	587	24.22808	644	25.37716
474	21.77154	531	23.04344	588	24.24871	645	25.39685
475	21.79449	532	23.06513	589	24.26932	646	25.41653
476	21.81742	533	23.08679	590	24.28992	647	25.43619
477	21.84033	534	23.10844	591	24.31049	648	25.45584
478	21.86321	535	23.13007	592	24.33105	649	25.47548
479	21.88607	536	23.15167	593	24.35159	650	25.49510
480	21.90890	537	23.17326	594	24.37212	651	25.51470
481	21.93171	538	23.19483	595	24.39262	652	25.53429
482	21.95450	539	23.21637	596	24.41311	653	25.55386
483	21.97726	540	23.23790	597	24.43358	654	25.57342
484	22.00000	541	23.25941	598	24.45404	655	25.59297
485	22.02272	542	23.28089	599	24.47448	656	25.61250
486	22.04541	543	23.30236	600	24.49490	657	25.63201
487	22.06808	544	23.32381	601	24.51530	658	25.65151
488	22.09072	545	23.34524	602	24.53569	659	25.67100
489	22.11334	546	23.36664	603	24.55606	660	25.69047
490	22.13594	547	23.38803	604	24.57641	661	25.70992
491	22.15852	548	23.40940	605	24.59675	662	25.72936
492	22.18107	549	23.43075	606	24.61707	663	25.74879
493	22.20360	550	23.45208	607	24.63737	664	25.76820
494	22.22611	551	23.47339	608	24.65766	665	25.78759
495	22.24860	552	23.49468	609	24.67793	666	25.80698
496	22.27106	553	23.51595	610	24.69818	667	25.82634
497	22.29350	554	23.53720	611	24.71841	668	25.84570
498	22.31591	555	23.55844	612	24.73863	669	25.86503
499	22.33831	556	23.57965	613	24.75884	670	25.88436
500	22.36068	557	23.60085	614	24.77902	671	25.90367
501	22.38303	558	23.62202	615	24.79919	672	25.92296
502	22.40536	559	23.64318	616	24.81935	673	25.94224
503	22.42766	560	23.66432	617	24.83948	674	25.96151
504	22.44994	561	23.68544	618	24.85961	675	25.98076
505	22.47221	562	23.70654	619	24.87971	676	26.00000
506	22.49444	563	23.72762	620	24.89980	677	26.01922
507	22.51666	564	23.74868	621	24.91987	678	26.03843
508	22.53886	565	23.76973	622	24.93993	679	26.05763
509	22.56103	566	23.79075	623	24.95997	680	26.07681
510	22.58318	567	23.81176	624	24.97999	681	26.09598
511	22.60531	568	23.83275	625	25.00000	682	26.11513
512	22.62742	569	23.85372	626	25.01999	683	26.13427
513	22.64950	570	23.87467	627	25.03997	684	26.15339

Appendix D—continued

n	√n	n	√n	n	√n	n	√n
685	26.17250	743	27.25803	801	28.30194	859	29.30870
686	26.19160	744	27.27636	802	28.31960	860	29.32576
687	26.21068	745	27.29469	803	28.33725	861	29.34280
688	26.22975	746	27.31300	804	28.35489	862	29.35984
689	26.24881	747	27.33130	805	28.37252	863	29.37686
690	26.26785	748	27.34959	806	28.39014	864	29.39388
691	26.28688	749	27.36786	807	28.40775	865	29.41088
692	26.30589	750	27.38613	808	28.42534	866	29.42788
693	26.32489	751	27.40438	809	28.44293	867	29.44486
694	26.34388	752	27.42262	810	28.46050	868	29.46184
695	26.36285	753	27.44085	811	28.47806	869	29.47881
696	26.38181	754	27.45906	812	28.49561	870	29.49576
697	26.40076	755	27.47726	813	28.51315	871	29.51271
698	26.41969	756	27.49545	814	28.53069	872	29.52965
699	26.43861	757	27.51363	815	28.54820	873	29.54657
700	26.45751	758	27.53180	816	28.56571	874	29.56349
701	26.47640	759	27.54995	817	28.58321	875	29.58040
702	26.49528	760	27.56810	818	28.60070	876	29.59730
703	26.51415	761	27.58623	819	28.61818	877	29.61419
704	26.53300	762	27.60435	820	28.63564	878	29.63106
705	26.55184	763	27.62245	821	28.65310	879	29.64793
706	26.57066	764	27.64055	822	28.67054	880	29.66479
707	26.58947	765	27.65863	823	28.68798	881	29.68164
708	26.60827	766	27.67671	824	28.70540	882	29.69848
709	26.62705	767	27.69476	825	28.72281	883	29.71532
710	26.64583	768	27.71281	826	28.74022	884	29.73214
711	26.66458	769	27.73085	827	28.75761	885	29.74895
712	26.68333	770	27.74887	828	28.77499	886	29.76575
713	26.70206	771	27.76689	829	28.79236	887	29.78255
714	26.72078	772	27.78489	830	28.80972	888	29.79333
715	26.73948	773	27.80288	831	28.82707	889	29.81610
716	26.75818	774	27.82086	832	28.84441	890	29.83287
717	26.77686	775	27.83882	833	28.86174	891	29.84962
718	26.79552	776	27.85678	834	28.87906	892	29.86637
719	26.81418	777	27.87472	835	28.89637	893	29.88311
720	26.83282	778	27.89265	836	28.91366	894	29.89983
721	26.85144	779	27.91057	837	28.93095	895	29.91655
722	26.87006	780	27.92848	838	28.94823	896	29.93326
723	26.88866	781	27.94638	839	28.96550	897	29.94996
724	26.90725	782	27.96426	840	28.98275	898	29.96665
725	26.92582	783	27.98214	841	29.00000	899	29.98333
726	26.94439	784	28.00000	842	29.01724	900	30.00000
727	26.96294	785	28.01785	843	29.03446	901	30.01666
728	26.98148	786	28.03569	844	29.05168	902	20.03331
729	27.00000	787	28.05352	845	29.06888	903	30.04996
730	27.01851	788	28.07134	846	29.08608	904	30.06659
731	27.03701	789	28.08914	847	29.10326	905	30.08322
732	27.05550	790	28.10694	848	29.12044	906	30.09983
733	27.07397	791	28.12472	849	29.13760	907	30.11644
734	27.09243	792	28.14249	850	29.15476	908	30.13304
735	27.11088	793	28.16026	851	29.17190	909	30.14963
736	27.12932	794	28.17801	852	29.18904	910	30.16621
737	27.14774	795	28.19574	853	29.20616	911	30.18278
738	27.16616	796	28.21347	854	29.22328	912	30.19934
739	27.18455	797	28.23119	855	29.24038	913	30.21589
740	27.20294	798	28.24889	856	29.25748	914	30.23243
741	27.22132	799	28.26659	857	29.27456	915	30.24897
742	27.23968	800	28.28472	858	29.29164	916	30.26549

Appendix D—continued

n	$\sqrt{n}$	n	$\sqrt{n}$	n	$\sqrt{n}$	n	$\sqrt{n}$
917	30.28201	938	30.62679	959	30.96773	980	31.30495
918	30.29851	939	30.64311	960	30.98387	981	31.32092
919	30.31501	940	30.65942	961	31.00000	982	31.33688
920	30.33150	941	30.67572	962	31.01612	983	31.35283
921	30.34798	942	30.69202	963	31.03224	984	31.36877
922	30.36445	943	30.70831	964	31.04835	985	31.38471
923	30.38092	944	30.72458	965	31.06445	986	31.40064
924	30.39737	945	30.74085	966	31.08054	987	31.41656
925	30.41381	946	30.75711	967	31.09662	988	31.43247
926	30.43025	947	30.77337	968	31.11270	989	31.44837
927	30.44667	948	30.78961	969	31.12876	990	31.46427
928	30.46309	949	30.80584	970	31.14482	991	31.48015
929	30.47950	950	30.82207	971	31.16087	992	31.49603
930	30.49590	951	30.83829	972	31.17691	993	31.51190
931	30.51229	952	30.85450	973	31.19295	994	31.52777
932	30.52868	953	30.87070	974	31.20897	995	31.54362
933	30.54505	954	30.88689	975	31.22499	996	31.55947
934	30.56141	955	30.90307	976	31.24100	997	31.57531
935	30.57777	956	30.91925	977	31.25700	998	31.59114
936	30.59412	957	30.93542	978	31.27299	999	31.60696
937	30.61046	958	30.95158	979	31.28898	1000	31.62278

Appendix E

Arcsin Transformation ($\phi = 2 \arcsin \sqrt{X}$)*

X	ϕ	X	ϕ	X	ϕ	X	ϕ	X	ϕ
.001	.0633	.041	.4078	.36	1.2870	.76	2.1177	.971	2.7993
.002	.0895	.042	.4128	.37	1.3078	.77	2.1412	.972	2.8053
.003	.1096	.043	.4178	.38	1.3284	.78	2.1652	.973	2.8115
.004	.1266	.044	.4227	.39	1.3490	.79	2.1895	.974	2.8177
.005	.1415	.045	.4275	.40	1.3694	.80	2.2143	.075	2.8240
.006	.1551	.046	.4323	.41	1.3898	.81	2.2395	.976	2.8305
.007	.1675	.047	.4371	.42	1.4101	.82	2.2653	.977	2.8371
.008	.1791	.048	.4418	.43	1.4303	.83	2.2916	.978	2.8438
.009	.1900	.049	.4464	.44	1.4505	.84	2.3186	.979	2.8507
.010	.2003	.050	.4510	.45	1.4706	.85	2.3462	.980	2.8578
.011	.2101	.06	.4949	.46	1.4907	.86	2.3746	.981	2.8650
.012	.2195	.07	.5355	.47	1.5108	.87	2.4039	.982	2.8725
.013	.2285	.08	.5735	.48	1.5308	.88	2.4341	.983	2.8801
.014	.2372	.09	.6094	.49	1.5508	.89	2.4655	.984	2.8879
.015	.2456	.10	.6435	.50	1.5708	.90	2.4981	.985	2.8960
.016	.2537	.11	.6761	.51	1.5908	.91	2.5322	.986	2.904
.017	.2615	.12	.7075	.52	1.6108	.92	2.5681	.987	2.9131
.018	.2691	.13	.7377	.53	1.6308	.93	2.6062	.988	2.9221
.019	.2766	.14	.7670	.54	1.6509	.94	2.6467	.989	2.9315
.020	.2838	.15	.7954	.55	1.6710	.95	2.6906	.990	2.941
.021	.2909	.16	.8230	.56	1.6911	.951	2.6952	.991	2.9516
.022	.2978	.17	.8500	.57	1.7113	.952	2.6998	.992	2.9625
.023	.3045	.18	.8763	.58	1.7315	.953	2.7045	.993	2.9741
.024	.3111	.19	.9021	.59	1.7518	.954	2.7093	.994	2.9865
.025	.3176	.20	.9273	.60	1.7722	.955	2.7141	.995	3.0001
.026	.3239	.21	.9521	.61	1.7926	.956	2.7189	.996	3.0150
.027	.3301	.22	.9764	.62	1.8132	.957	2.7238	.997	3.0320
.028	.3363	.23	1.0004	.63	1.8338	.958	2.7288	.998	3.0521
.029	.3423	.24	1.0239	.64	1.8546	.959	2.7338	.999	3.0783
.030	.3482	.25	1.0472	.65	1.8755	.960	2.7389		
.031	.3540	.26	1.0701	.66	1.8965	.961	2.7440		
.032	.3597	.27	1.0928	.67	1.9177	.962	2.7492		
.033	.3654	.28	1.1152	.68	1.9391	.963	2.7545		
.034	.3709	.29	1.1374	.69	1.9606	.964	2.7598		
.035	.3764	.30	1.1593	.70	1.9823	.965	2.7652		
.036	.3818	.31	1.1810	.71	2.0042	.966	2.7707		
.037	.3871	.32	1.2025	.72	2.0264	.967	2.7762		
.038	.3924	.33	1.2239	.73	2.0488	.968	2.7819		
.039	.3976	.34	1.2451	.74	2.0715	.869	2.7876		
.040	.4027	.35	1.2661	.75	2.0944	.970	2.7934		

* This table is reproduced from Table B-5 in Winer, B., *Statistical Principles in Experimental Design*, 1971, by permission of McGraw-Hill Co.

Appendix F

z Values (Normal Curve)*

z	.00	.01	.02	.03	.04	.05	.06	.07	.08	.09
0.0	.0000	.0040	.0080	.0120	.0160	.0199	.0239	.0279	.0319	.0359
0.1	.0398	.0438	.0478	.0517	.0557	.0596	.0636	.0675	.0714	.0753
0.2	.0793	.0832	.0871	.0910	.0948	.0987	.1026	.1064	.1103	.1141
0.3	.1179	.1217	.1255	.1293	.1331	.1368	.1406	.1443	.1480	.1517
0.4	.1554	.1591	.1628	.1664	.1700	.1736	.1772	.1808	.1844	.1879
0.5	.1915	.1950	.1985	.2019	.2054	.2088	.2123	.2157	.2190	.2224
0.6	.2257	.2291	.2324	.2357	.2389	.2422	.2454	.2486	.2517	.2549
0.7	.2580	.2611	.2642	.2673	.2704	.2734	.2764	.2794	.2823	.2852
0.8	.2881	.2910	.2939	.2967	.2995	.3023	.3051	.3078	.3106	.3133
0.9	.3159	.3186	.3212	.3238	.3264	.3289	.3315	.3340	.3365	.3389
1.0	.3413	.3438	.3461	.3485	.3508	.3531	.3554	.3577	.3599	.3621
1.1	.3643	.3665	.3686	.3708	.3729	.3749	.3770	.3790	.3810	.3830
1.2	.3849	.3869	.3888	.3907	.3925	.3944	.3962	.3980	.3997	.4015
1.3	.4032	.4049	.4066	.4082	.4099	.4115	.4131	.4147	.4162	.4177
1.4	.4192	.4207	.4222	.4236	.4251	.4265	.4279	.4292	.4306	.4319
1.5	.4332	.4345	.4357	.4370	.4382	.4394	.4406	.4418	.4429	.4441
1.6	.4452	.4463	.4474	.4484	.4495	.4505	.4515	.4525	.4535	.4545
1.7	.4554	.4564	.4573	.4582	.4591	.4599	.4608	.4616	.4625	.4633
1.8	.4641	.4649	.4656	.4664	.4671	.4678	.4686	.4693	.4699	.4706
1.9	.4713	.4719	.4726	.4732	.4738	.4744	.4750	.4756	.4761	.4767
2.0	.4772	.4778	.4783	.4788	.4793	.4798	.4803	.4808	.4812	.4817
2.1	.4821	.4826	.4830	.4834	.4838	.4842	.4846	.4850	.4854	.4857
2.2	.4861	.4864	.4868	.4871	.4875	.4878	.4881	.4884	.4887	.4890
2.3	.4893	.4896	.4898	.4901	.4904	.4906	.4909	.4911	.4913	.4916
2.4	.4918	.4920	.4922	.4925	.4927	.4929	.4931	.4932	.4934	.4336
2.5	.4938	.4940	.4941	.4943	.4945	.4946	.4948	.4949	.4951	.4952
2.6	.4953	.4955	.4956	.4957	.4959	.4960	.4961	.4962	.4963	.4964
2.7	.4965	.4966	.4967	.4968	.4969	.4970	.4971	.4972	.4973	.4974
2.8	.4974	.4975	.4976	.4977	.4977	.4978	.4979	.4979	.4980	.4981
2.9	.4981	.4982	.4982	.4983	.4984	.4984	.4985	.4985	.4986	.4986
3.0	.4987	.4987	.4987	.4988	.4988	.4989	.4989	.4989	.4990	.4990
3.1	.49903									
3.2	.49931									
3.3	.49952									
3.4	.49966									
3.5	.49977									
3.6	.49984									
3.7	.49989									
3.8	.49993									
3.9	.49995									
4.0	.50000									

* The table of Z scores is not really necessary, because so few values are needed for the determination of probability. Also, the degrees of freedom are, in a sense, built into the formula and are not a part of the final probability consideration.

If the z score equals or exceeds this value:	The result is significant at this level of confidence:
1.96	.05
2.33	.02
2.58	.01
3.33	.001

Appendix G

Critical Values for the F Distribution*

Degrees of Freedom for the Numerator = 2

df for the Denominator	Probability Level				
	.05	.02	.01	.002	.001
2.	19.000	49.000	99.000	498.992	998.956
3.	9.552	18.858	30.816	92.993	148.495
4.	6.944	12.142	18.000	42.721	61.244
5.	5.786	9.454	13.274	27.528	37.122
6.	5.143	8.052	10.925	20.811	27.000
7.	4.737	7.203	9.547	17.163	21.689
8.	4.459	6.637	8.649	14.915	18.493
9.	4.256	6.234	8.021	13.405	16.387
10.	4.103	5.934	7.559	12.329	14.905
11.	3.982	5.701	7.206	11.525	13.811
12.	3.885	5.516	6.927	10.904	12.974
13.	3.806	5.366	6.701	10.410	12.313
14.	3.739	5.241	6.515	10.008	11.779
15.	3.682	5.135	6.359	9.676	11.339
16.	3.634	5.046	6.226	9.396	10.971
17.	3.592	4.968	6.112	9.158	10.658
18.	3.555	4.900	6.013	8.953	10.390
19.	3.522	4.840	5.926	8.774	10.157
20.	3.493	4.788	5.849	8.616	9.953
21.	3.467	4.740	5.780	8.477	9.772
22.	3.443	4.698	5.719	8.353	9.612
23.	3.422	4.660	5.664	8.242	9.468
24.	3.403	4.625	5.614	8.142	9.339
25.	3.385	4.593	5.568	8.051	9.222
26.	3.369	4.564	5.526	7.968	9.116
27.	3.354	4.538	5.488	7.892	9.019
28.	3.340	4.513	5.453	7.823	8.930
29.	3.328	4.491	5.420	7.759	8.849
30.	3.316	4.470	5.390	7.700	8.773
31.	3.305	4.450	5.362	7.645	8.704
32.	3.295	4.432	5.336	7.594	8.639
33.	3.285	4.415	5.312	7.547	8.578
34.	3.276	4.399	5.289	7.503	8.522
35.	3.267	4.384	5.268	7.461	8.470
36.	3.259	4.370	5.248	7.422	8.420
37.	3.252	4.356	5.229	7.386	8.374
38.	3.245	4.344	5.211	7.351	8.330
39.	3.238	4.332	5.194	7.319	8.289
40.	3.232	4.321	5.179	7.288	8.251
50.	3.183	4.235	5.057	7.055	7.956
60.	3.150	4.179	4.977	6.905	7.768
70.	3.128	4.139	4.922	6.800	7.637
80.	3.111	4.110	4.881	6.723	7.540
90.	3.098	4.087	4.849	6.664	7.466
100.	3.087	4.069	4.824	6.617	7.408

* The values for this table were generated by computer, using a FORTRAN (MDFI) program.

Degrees of Freedom for the Numerator = 3

df for the Denominator	Probability Level				
	.05	.02	.01	.002	.001
2.	19.164	49.166	99.166	499.158	999.121
3.	9.276	18.109	29.461	88.469	141.006
4.	6.591	11.344	16.693	39.262	56.173
5.	5.410	8.670	12.060	24.701	33.202
6.	4.757	7.287	9.779	18.345	23.703
7.	4.347	6.454	8.451	14.927	18.772
8.	4.066	5.901	7.591	12.837	15.830
9.	3.863	5.510	6.992	11.441	13.902
10.	3.708	5.218	6.552	10.451	12.552
11.	3.588	4.993	6.217	9.714	11.561
12.	3.490	4.814	5.952	9.146	10.804
13.	3.411	4.669	5.740	8.696	10.209
14.	3.344	4.549	5.564	8.331	9.729
15.	3.287	4.447	5.417	8.030	9.335
16.	3.239	4.361	5.292	7.777	9.006
17.	3.197	4.286	5.185	7.561	8.727
18.	3.160	4.221	5.092	7.376	8.488
19.	3.127	4.164	5.010	7.214	8.280
20.	3.098	4.113	4.938	7.073	8.098
21.	3.072	4.068	4.874	6.947	7.938
22.	3.049	4.028	4.817	6.836	7.796
23.	3.028	3.991	4.765	6.736	7.669
24.	3.009	3.958	4.718	6.646	7.555
25.	2.991	3.928	4.676	6.565	7.451
26.	2.975	3.900	4.637	6.490	7.357
27.	2.960	3.874	4.601	6.422	7.272
28.	2.947	3.851	4.568	6.360	7.193
29.	2.934	3.829	4.538	6.303	7.121
30.	2.922	3.809	4.510	6.250	7.054
31.	2.911	3.791	4.484	6.201	6.993
32.	2.901	3.773	4.459	6.156	6.936
33.	2.892	3.757	4.437	6.114	6.883
34.	2.883	3.742	4.416	6.074	6.833
35.	2.874	3.727	4.396	6.037	6.787
36.	2.866	3.714	4.377	6.003	6.744
37.	2.859	3.701	4.360	5.970	6.703
38.	2.852	3.689	4.343	5.939	6.665
39.	2.845	3.678	4.327	5.910	6.629
40.	2.839	3.667	4.313	5.883	6.595
50.	2.790	3.585	4.199	5.676	6.336
60.	2.758	3.532	4.126	5.542	6.171
70.	2.736	3.494	4.074	5.450	6.057
80.	2.719	3.467	4.036	5.381	5.972
90.	2.706	3.445	4.007	5.329	5.908
100.	2.695	3.428	3.984	5.287	5.857

Degrees of Freedom for the Numerator = 4

df for the Denominator	Probability Level				
	.05	.02	.01	.002	.001
2.	19.247	49.249	99.249	499.242	999.206
3.	9.117	17.697	28.709	86.014	37.124
4.	6.388	10.899	15.976	37.381	53.454
5.	5.192	8.233	11.391	23.164	31.085
6.	4.534	6.860	9.149	17.008	21.925
7.	4.120	6.035	7.847	13.716	17.199
8.	3.838	5.489	7.006	11.710	14.391
9.	3.633	5.103	6.422	10.376	12.560
10.	3.478	4.816	5.994	9.432	11.283
11.	3.357	4.594	5.668	8.731	10.346
12.	3.259	4.419	5.412	8.192	9.633
13.	3.179	4.276	5.205	7.766	9.073
14.	3.112	4.158	5.035	7.420	8.623
15.	3.056	4.058	4.893	7.135	8.253
16.	3.007	3.974	4.772	6.896	7.944
17.	2.965	3.901	4.669	6.693	7.683
18.	2.928	3.837	4.579	6.518	7.459
19.	2.895	3.781	4.500	6.366	7.265
20.	2.866	3.731	4.431	6.232	7.096
21.	2.840	3.687	4.369	6.115	6.947
22.	2.817	3.647	4.313	6.010	6.814
23.	2.796	3.611	4.263	5.916	6.696
24.	2.776	3.579	4.219	5.832	6.589
25.	2.759	3.549	4.177	5.755	6.493
26.	2.743	3.522	4.140	5.685	6.406
27.	2.728	3.497	4.106	5.622	6.326
28.	2.714	3.475	4.074	5.564	6.253
29.	2.701	3.454	4.045	5.510	6.186
30.	2.690	3.434	4.018	5.460	6.124
31.	2.679	3.416	3.993	5.415	6.067
32.	2.669	3.399	3.969	5.372	6.014
33.	2.659	3.383	3.948	5.333	5.965
34.	2.650	3.354	3.927	5.296	5.919
35.	2.641	3.341	3.908	5.261	5.877
36.	2.633	3.328	3.890	5.229	5.836
37.	2.626	3.317	3.874	5.198	5.799
38.	2.619	3.306	3.858	5.170	5.763
39.	2.612	3.295	3.842	5.143	5.730
40.	2.606	3.295	3.828	5.117	5.698
50.	2.557	3.215	3.720	4.923	5.459
60.	2.525	3.163	3.649	4.799	5.307
70.	2.503	3.127	3.600	4.712	5.201
80.	2.486	3.100	3.563	4.649	5.123
90.	2.473	3.079	3.535	4.600	5.064
100.	2.463	3.062	3.513	4.561	5.017

Degrees of Freedom for the Numerator = 5

df for the Denominator	Probability Level				
	.05	.02	.01	.002	.001
2.	19.296	49.299	99.299	499.292	999.255
3.	9.013	17.425	28.239	84.420	134.758
4.	6.256	10.616	15.520	36.213	51.708
5.	5.050	7.952	10.967	22.194	29.746
6.	4.387	6.585	8.745	16.162	20.801
7.	3.972	5.765	7.460	12.951	16.205
8.	3.687	5.223	6.632	10.998	13.484
9.	3.482	4.839	6.057	9.701	11.713
10.	3.326	4.555	5.636	8.786	10.480
11.	3.204	4.336	5.316	8.107	9.578
12.	3.106	4.162	5.064	7.586	8.892
13.	3.025	4.020	4.861	7.174	8.354
14.	2.958	3.904	4.695	6.841	7.922
15.	2.901	3.805	4.556	6.567	7.567
16.	2.852	3.721	4.438	6.336	7.272
17.	2.810	3.649	4.336	6.140	7.022
18.	2.773	3.586	4.248	5.972	6.808
19.	2.740	3.531	4.171	5.826	6.622
20.	2.711	3.482	4.103	5.698	6.460
21.	2.685	3.438	4.042	5.584	6.318
22.	2.661	3.399	3.988	5.484	6.191
23.	2.640	3.363	3.939	5.394	6.078
24.	2.621	3.331	3.895	5.313	5.977
25.	2.603	3.302	3.855	5.239	5.885
26.	2.587	3.275	3.818	5.172	5.802
27.	2.572	3.251	3.785	5.111	5.726
28.	2.558	3.228	3.754	5.055	5.657
29.	2.545	3.207	3.725	5.004	5.593
30.	2.534	3.188	3.699	4.957	5.534
31.	2.522	3.170	3.675	4.913	5.479
32.	2.512	3.153	3.652	4.872	5.429
33.	2.503	3.137	3.630	4.834	5.382
34.	2.494	3.123	3.611	4.799	5.338
35.	2.485	3.109	3.592	4.766	5.298
36.	2.477	3.096	3.574	4.734	5.259
37.	2.470	3.084	3.558	4.706	5.224
38.	2.463	3.072	3.542	4.678	5.190
39.	2.456	3.061	3.528	4.652	5.158
40.	2.449	3.051	3.514	4.628	5.128
50.	2.400	2.972	3.408	4.442	4.901
60.	2.368	2.921	3.339	4.324	4.756
70.	2.346	2.885	3.291	4.241	4.656
80.	2.329	2.858	3.255	4.180	4.582
90.	2.316	2.837	3.228	4.133	4.526
100.	2.305	2.821	3.206	4.097	4.481

Degrees of Freedom for the Numerator = 6

df for the Denominator	Probability Level				
	.05	.02	.01	.002	.001
2.	19.329	49.332	99.332	499.323	999.284
3.	8.942	17.246	27.907	83.413	132.947
4.	6.163	10.418	15.206	35.397	50.523
5.	4.950	7.757	10.673	21.526	28.840
6.	4.284	6.393	8.466	15.581	20.029
7.	3.866	5.575	7.192	12.420	15.522
8.	3.581	5.036	6.371	10.503	12.858
9.	3.374	4.655	5.802	9.234	11.128
10.	3.217	4.371	5.386	8.337	9.925
11.	3.095	4.153	5.069	7.674	9.046
12.	2.996	3.980	4.820	7.166	8.379
13.	2.915	3.840	4.620	6.764	7.856
14.	2.848	3.724	4.456	6.439	7.436
15.	2.791	3.626	4.318	6.170	7.092
16.	2.741	3.543	4.202	5.946	6.805
17.	2.699	3.471	4.102	5.755	6.563
18.	2.661	3.408	4.015	5.592	6.355
19.	2.628	3.353	3.938	5.449	6.175
20.	2.599	3.304	3.871	5.325	6.018
21.	2.573	3.261	3.812	5.214	5.880
22.	2.549	3.222	3.758	5.117	5.758
23.	2.528	3.187	3.710	5.029	5.649
24.	2.508	3.155	3.667	4.950	5.550
25.	2.490	3.126	3.627	4.879	5.462
26.	2.474	3.099	3.591	4.814	5.381
27.	2.459	3.075	3.558	4.755	5.308
28.	2.445	3.052	3.527	4.700	5.241
29.	2.432	3,032	3.499	4.651	5.179
30.	2.421	3.012	3.473	4.604	5.122
31.	2.409	2.994	3.449	4.562	5.070
32.	2.399	2.978	3.427	4.522	5.021
33.	2.389	2.962	3.406	4.485	4.976
34.	2.380	2.948	3.386	4.451	4.933
35.	2.372	2.934	3.368	4.419	4.894
36.	2.364	2.921	3.351	4.389	4.857
37.	2.356	2.909	3.335	4.360	4.823
38.	2.349	2.898	3.319	4.334	4.790
39.	2.342	2.887	3.305	4.309	4.759
40.	2.336	2.877	3.291	4.285	4.731
50.	2.286	2.798	3.186	4.105	4.512
60.	2.254	2.747	3.119	3.990	4.372
70.	2.231	2.711	3.071	3.910	4.275
80.	2.214	2.685	3.036	3.851	4.204
90.	2.201	2.664	3.009	3.806	4.150
100.	2.191	2.648	2.988	3.770	4.107

Degrees of Freedom for the Numerator = 7

df for the Denominator	Probability Level				
	.05	.02	.01	.002	.001
2.	19.353	49.356	99.356	499.349	999.311
3.	8.886	17.109	27.672	82.546	131.745
4.	6.094	10.272	14.977	34.808	4.9662
5.	4.876	7.613	10.457	21.043	28.155
6.	4.207	6.251	8.260	15.154	19.463
7.	3.787	5.436	6.993	12.030	15.018
8.	3.500	4.897	6.178	10.141	12.397
9.	3.293	4.517	5.613	8.890	10.698
10.	3.135	4.235	5.200	8.008	9.517
11.	3.012	4.018	4.886	7.355	8.655
12.	2.913	3.845	4.640	6.855	8.001
13.	2.832	3.705	4.441	6.460	7.488
14.	2.764	3.589	4.278	6.141	7.077
15.	2.707	3.492	4.142	5.878	6.741
16.	2.657	3.409	4.026	5.657	6.460
17.	2.614	3.337	3.927	5.471	6.223
18.	2.577	3.275	3.841	5.310	6.021
19.	2.543	3.220	3.765	5.170	5.845
20.	2.514	3.171	3.699	5.048	5.692
21.	2.488	3.128	3.640	4.940	5.557
22.	2.464	3.089	3.587	4.844	5.438
23.	2.442	3.054	3.539	4.759	5.331
24.	2.423	3.022	3.496	4.681	5.235
25.	2.405	2.993	3.457	4.611	5.148
26.	2.388	2.967	3.421	4.548	5.070
27.	2.373	2.943	3.388	4.490	4.998
28.	2.359	2.920	3.358	4.437	4.933
29.	2.346	2.899	3.330	4.388	4.873
30.	2.334	2.880	3.304	4.343	4.817
31.	2.323	2.862	3.281	4.301	4.766
32.	2.313	2.846	3.258	4.262	4.719
33.	2.303	2.830	3.238	4.226	4.675
34.	2.294	2.816	3.218	4.193	4.633
35.	2.285	2.802	3.200	4.161	4.595
36.	2.277	2.789	3.183	4.131	4.559
37.	2.270	2.777	3.167	4.104	4.525
38.	2.262	2.766	3.152	4.078	4.494
39.	2.255	2.755	3.137	4.053	4.464
40.	2.249	2.745	3.124	4.030	4.435
50.	2.199	2.667	3.020	3.854	4.222
60.	2.166	2.616	2.953	3.742	4.086
70.	2.143	2.580	2.906	3.663	3.992
80.	2.126	2.553	2.871	3.606	3.923
90.	2.113	2.533	2.845	3.562	3.870
100.	2.102	2.517	2.823	3.527	3.829

Degrees of Freedom for the Numerator = 8

df for the Denominator	Probability Level				
	.05	.02	.01	.002	.001
2.	19.371	49.373	99.374	499.366	999.327
3.	8.845	17.012	27.505	81.957	130.697
4.	6.041	10.161	14.801	34.341	48.961
5.	4.819	7.503	10.290	20.669	27.653
6.	4.147	6.141	8.102	14.827	19.033
7.	3.726	5.327	6.840	11.732	14.634
8.	3.438	4.790	6.029	9.862	12.046
9.	3.229	4.410	5.467	8.625	10.367
10.	3.072	4.129	5.057	7.754	9.204
11.	2.948	3.912	4.744	7.110	8.355
12.	2.848	3.740	4.499	6.616	7.710
13.	2.767	3.600	4.302	6.226	7.206
14.	2.699	3.485	4.140	5.911	6.801
15.	2.641	3.387	4.005	5.652	6.471
16.	2.591	3.304	3.890	5.435	6.195
17.	2.548	3.233	3.791	5.251	5.962
18.	2.510	3.171	3.706	5.093	5.763
19.	2.477	3.116	3.631	4.955	5.590
20.	2.447	3.067	3.564	4.835	5.440
21.	2.420	3.024	3.506	4.728	5.308
22.	2.397	2.985	3.453	4.634	5.190
23.	2.375	2.950	3.406	4.549	5.085
24.	2.355	2.919	3.363	4.473	4.991
25.	2.337	2.890	3.324	4.404	4.906
26.	2.321	2.863	3.288	4.342	4.829
27.	2.305	2.839	3.256	4.285	4.759
28.	2.291	2.817	3.226	4.232	4.695
29.	2.278	2.796	3.198	4.184	4.636
30.	2.266	2.777	3.173	4.140	4.581
31.	2.255	2.759	3.149	4.099	4.531
32.	2.244	2.742	3.127	4.061	4.485
33.	2.235	2.727	3.106	4.025	4.441
34.	2.225	2.712	3.087	3.992	4.401
35.	2.217	2.699	3.069	3.961	4.363
36.	2.209	2.686	3.052	3.932	4.328
37.	2.201	2.674	3.036	3.905	4.295
38.	2.194	2.662	3.021	3.879	4.264
39.	2.187	2.651	3.006	3.855	4.235
40.	2.180	2.641	2.993	3.832	4.207
50.	2.130	2.563	2.890	3.659	3.998
60.	2.097	2.512	2.823	3.548	3.865
70.	2.074	2.476	2.777	3.471	3.773
80.	2.056	2.450	2.742	3.415	3.705
90.	2.043	2.429	2.715	3.371	3.653
100.	2.032	2.413	2.694	3.337	3.612

Degrees of Freedom for the Numerator = 9

df for the Denominator	Probability Level				
	.05	.02	.01	.002	.001
2.	19.385	49.387	99.387	499.377	999.337
3.	8.813	16.929	27.336	81.638	130.087
4.	5.999	10.073	14.659	34.005	48.468
5.	4.772	7.416	10.158	20.375	27.248
6.	4.099	6.054	7.976	14.570	18.687
7.	3.676	5.241	6.719	11.497	14.332
8.	3.388	4.705	5.911	9.642	11.765
9.	3.179	4.325	5.351	8.415	10.107
10.	3.020	4.044	4.943	7.553	8.956
11.	2.896	3.827	4.632	6.915	8.116
12.	2.796	3.656	4.387	6.426	7.479
13.	2.714	3.516	4.191	6.040	6.982
14.	2.646	3.401	4.030	5.729	6.583
15.	2.588	3.303	3.895	5.473	6.256
16.	2.538	3.221	3.780	5.258	5.984
17.	2.494	3.149	3.682	5.076	5.754
18.	2.456	3.087	3.597	4.919	5.557
19.	2.423	3.032	3.523	4.783	5.388
20.	2.393	2.984	3.457	4.664	5.239
21.	2.366	2.940	3.398	4.559	5.109
22.	2.342	2.902	3.346	4.466	4.993
23.	2.320	2.867	3.299	4.382	4.890
24.	2.300	2.835	3.256	4.307	4.797
25.	2.282	2.806	3.217	4.239	4.713
26.	2.265	2.780	3.182	4.177	4.637
27.	2.250	2.755	3.149	4.121	4.568
28.	2.236	2.733	3.120	4.069	4.505
29.	2.223	2.712	3.092	4.021	4.447
30.	2.211	2.693	3.066	3.978	4.393
31.	2.199	2.675	3.043	3.937	4.343
32.	2.189	2.659	3.021	3.899	4.298
33.	2.179	2.643	3.000	3.864	4.255
34.	2.170	2.629	2.981	3.832	4.215
35.	2.161	2.615	2.963	3.801	4.178
36.	2.153	2.602	2.946	3.772	4.144
37.	2.145	2.590	2.930	3.745	4.111
38.	2.137	2.579	2.915	3.720	4.080
39.	2.131	2.568	2.901	3.696	4.051
40.	2.124	2.558	2.888	3.674	4.024
50.	2.073	2.479	2.785	3.503	3.818
60.	2.040	2.428	2.718	3.393	3.687
70.	2.017	2.392	2.672	3.317	3.597
80.	1.999	2.366	2.637	3.261	3.530
90.	1.986	2.345	2.611	3.218	3.479
100.	1.975	2.329	2.590	3.184	3.439

Degrees of Freedom for the Numerator = 10

df for the Denominator	Probability Level				
	.05	.02	.01	.002	.001
2.	19.396	49.398	99.399	499.391	999.352
3.	8.787	16.863	27.217	81.111	129.474
4.	5.965	10.005	14.550	33.711	48.011
5.	4.735	7.344	10.052	20.128	26.909
6.	4.060	5.984	7.874	14.360	18.410
7.	3.637	5.171	6.620	11.304	14.082
8.	3.347	4.635	5.814	9.463	11.541
9.	3.137	4.256	5.257	8.245	9.894
10.	2.978	3.975	4.849	7.389	8.753
11.	2.854	3.758	4.539	6.756	7.922
12.	2.753	3.587	4.296	6.271	7.292
13.	2.671	3.447	4.100	5.889	6.799
14.	2.602	3.332	3.939	5.580	6.404
15.	2.544	3.235	3.805	5.326	6.081
16.	2.494	3.152	3.691	5.113	5.812
17.	2.450	3.080	3.593	4.932	5.584
18.	2.412	3.018	3.508	4.777	5.390
19.	2.378	2.963	3.434	4.643	5.222
20.	2.348	2.915	3.368	4.525	5.075
21.	2.321	2.872	3.310	4.421	4.946
22.	2.297	2.833	3.258	4.328	4.832
23.	2.275	2.798	3.211	4.245	4.730
24.	2.255	2.766	3.168	4.171	4.638
25.	2.236	2.737	3.129	4.103	4.555
26.	2.220	2.711	3.094	4.042	4.480
27.	2.204	2.686	3.062	3.986	4.412
28.	2.190	2.664	3.032	3.935	4.349
29.	2.177	2.643	3.005	3.888	4.292
30.	2.165	2.624	2.979	3.844	4.239
31.	2.153	2.606	2.955	3.804	4.190
32.	2.142	2.589	2.934	3.767	4.145
33.	2.132	2.574	2.913	3.732	4.103
34.	2.123	2.559	2.894	3.700	4.063
35.	2.114	2.546	2.876	3.669	4.027
36.	2.106	2.533	2.859	3.641	3.992
37.	2.098	2.521	2.843	3.614	3.960
38.	2.091	2.509	2.828	3.589	3.930
39.	2.084	2.498	2.814	3.566	3.901
40.	2.077	2.488	2.801	3.543	3.874
50.	2.026	2.410	2.698	3.374	3.671
60.	1.993	2.359	2.632	3.266	3.541
70.	1.969	2.323	2.585	3.190	3.452
80.	1.951	2.296	2.551	3.135	3.386
90.	1.938	2.275	2.524	3.092	3.336
100.	1.927	2.259	2.503	3.059	3.296

Degrees of Freedom for the Numerator = 11

df for the Denominator	Probability Level				
	.05	.02	.01	.002	.001
2.	19.405	49.408	99.408	499.402	99.366
3.	8.761	16.807	27.120	80.786	128.777
4.	5.935	9.942	14.452	33.464	47.732
5.	4.704	7.284	9.963	19.942	26.639
6.	4.027	5.925	7.790	14.186	18.185
7.	3.603	5.112	6.539	11.146	13.877
8.	3.313	4.577	5.734	9.314	11.353
9.	3.102	4.198	5.178	8.104	9.717
10.	2.943	3.917	4.771	7.253	8.586
11.	2.818	3.701	4.462	6.624	7.761
12.	2.717	3.529	4.220	6.143	7.136
13.	2.635	3.390	4.024	5.763	6.648
14.	2.565	3.274	3.864	5.456	6.256
15.	2.507	3.177	3.730	5.204	5.935
16.	2.456	3.094	3.616	4.993	5.669
17.	2.413	3.022	3.519	4.813	5.443
18.	2.374	2.960	3.434	4.659	5.251
19.	2.340	2.905	3.360	4.526	5.084
20.	2.310	2.857	3.294	4.408	4.938
21.	2.283	2.814	3.236	4.305	4.811
22.	2.259	2.775	3.184	4.213	4.697
23.	2.236	2.740	3.137	4.131	4.596
24.	2.216	2.708	3.094	4.057	4.505
25.	2.198	2.679	3.056	3.990	4.423
26.	2.181	2.652	3.020	3.929	4.349
27.	2.166	2.628	2.988	3.874	4.281
28.	2.151	2.606	2.959	3.823	4.219
29.	2.138	2.585	2.931	3.776	4.162
30.	2.126	2.566	2.906	3.733	4.110
31.	2.114	2.548	2.882	3.693	4.061
32.	2.103	2.531	2.860	3.656	4.017
33.	2.093	2.515	2.840	3.622	3.975
34.	2.084	2.501	2.821	3.589	3.936
35.	2.075	2.487	2.803	3.559	3.900
36.	2.067	2.474	2.786	3.531	3.866
37.	2.059	2.462	2.770	3.505	3.834
38.	2.051	2.451	2.755	3.480	3.804
39.	2.044	2.440	2.741	3.456	3.776
40.	2.038	2.430	2.727	3.434	3.749
50.	1.986	2.351	2.625	3.266	3.548
60.	1.952	2.300	2.559	3.159	3.419
70.	1.928	2.264	2.512	3.084	3.331
80.	1.911	2.237	2.478	3.029	3.265
90.	1.897	2.216	2.451	2.987	3.215
100.	1.886	2.200	2.430	2.953	3.176

Degrees of Freedom for the Numerator = 12

df for the Denomina-tor	Probability Level				
	.05	.02	.01	.002	.001
2.	19.412	49.415	99.415	499.408	999.370
3.	8.745	16.755	27.034	80.659	128.252
4.	5.911	9.891	14.372	33.249	47.416
5.	4.677	7.235	9.890	19.773	26.420
6.	4.000	5.876	7.718	14.041	17.987
7.	3.575	5.064	6.469	11.014	13.705
8.	3.284	4.527	5.667	9.188	11.195
9.	3.073	4.149	5.112	7.986	9.571
10.	2.913	3.868	4.706	7.138	8.444
11.	2.788	3.652	4.398	6.513	7.626
12.	2.687	3.480	4.155	6.034	7.004
13.	2.604	3.341	3.960	5.656	6.519
14.	2.534	3.225	3.800	5.351	6.130
15.	2.475	3.128	3.666	5.101	5.812
16.	2.425	3.045	3.553	4.891	5.547
17.	2.381	2.974	3.455	4.712	5.324
18.	2.342	2.911	3.371	4.559	5.133
19.	2.308	2.856	3.296	4.426	4.967
20.	2.278	2.808	3.231	4.310	4.823
21.	2.250	2.764	3.173	4.207	4.696
22.	2.226	2.725	3.121	4.116	4.583
23.	2.204	2.690	3.074	4.034	4.483
24.	2.183	2.658	3.032	3.961	4.393
25.	2.165	2.630	2.993	3.894	4.312
26.	2.148	2.603	2.958	3.834	4.238
27.	2.132	2.579	2.926	3.779	4.170
28.	2.118	2.556	2.896	3.728	4.109
29.	2.104	2.535	2.869	3.682	4.053
30.	2.092	2.516	2.843	3.639	4.001
31.	2.080	2.498	2.820	3.599	3.953
32.	2.070	2.481	2.798	3.562	3.908
33.	2.059	2.466	2.777	3.528	3.867
34.	2.050	2.451	2.758	3.496	3.828
35.	2.041	2.437	2.740	3.466	3.792
36.	2.033	2.424	2.723	3.438	3.758
37.	2.025	2.412	2.707	3.412	3.727
38.	2.017	2.401	2.692	3.387	3.697
39.	2.010	2.390	2.678	3.364	3.669
40.	2.003	2.380	2.665	3.342	3.643
50.	1.952	2.301	2.563	3.174	3.443
60.	1.917	2.249	2.496	3.067	3.315
70.	1.893	2.213	2.450	2.993	3.227
80.	1.875	2.186	2.415	2.938	3.162
90.	1.861	2.165	2.389	2.896	3.113
100.	1.850	2.149	2.368	2.863	3.074

Degrees of Freedom for the Numerator = 13

df for the Denomina- tor	Probability Level				
	.05	.02	.01	.002	.001
2.	19.419	49.421	99.421	499.410	999.368
3.	8.726	16.715	26.995	80.429	128.481
4.	5.890	9.854	14.310	33.106	47.195
5.	4.655	7.193	9.827	19.628	26.218
6.	3.976	5.833	7.657	13.911	17.820
7.	3.550	5.022	6.410	10.898	13.563
8.	3.259	4.485	5.609	9.083	11.059
9.	3.048	4.107	5.055	7.884	9.443
10.	2.887	3.826	4.649	7.040	8.325
11.	2.761	3.610	4.342	6.417	7.510
12.	2.660	3.438	4.100	5.941	6.892
13.	2.577	3.299	3.905	5.565	6.410
14.	2.507	3.183	3.745	5.262	6.023
15.	2.448	3.086	3.611	5.012	5.707
16.	2.397	3.003	3.498	4.803	5.443
17.	2.353	2.931	3.401	4.625	5.221
18.	2.314	2.869	3.316	4.473	5.031
19.	2.280	2.814	3.242	4.341	4.867
20.	2.249	2.765	3.177	4.225	4.724
21.	2.222	2.722	3.119	4.123	4.598
22.	2.197	2.683	3.067	4.032	4.485
23.	2.175	2.648	3.020	3.951	4.386
24.	2.155	2.616	2.978	3.878	4.296
25.	2.136	2.587	2.939	3.811	4.215
26.	2.119	2.560	2.904	3.751	4.142
27.	2.103	2.536	2.871	3.696	4.076
28.	2.089	2.513	2.842	3.646	4.014
29.	2.075	2.492	2.814	3.600	3.958
30.	2.063	2.473	2.789	3.557	3.906
31.	2.051	2.455	2.766	3.518	3.859
32.	2.040	2.438	2.744	3.481	3.814
33.	2.030	2.422	2.723	3.447	3.773
34.	2.021	2.408	2.704	3.415	3.735
35.	2.012	2.394	2.686	3.385	3.699
36.	2.003	2.381	2.669	3.357	3.666
37.	1.995	2.369	2.653	3.331	3.634
38.	1.988	2.357	2.638	3.307	3.605
39.	1.981	2.346	2.624	3.283	3.577
40.	1.974	2.336	2.611	3.262	3.551
50.	1.921	2.257	2.508	3.095	3.352
60.	1.887	2.205	2.442	2.989	3.225
70.	1.863	2.169	2.395	2.914	3.138
80.	1.845	2.142	2.361	2.860	3.074
90.	1.830	2.121	2.334	2.818	3.024
100.	1.819	2.105	2.313	2.785	2.985

Degrees of Freedom for the Numerator = 14

df for the Denomina-tor	Probability Level				
	.05	.02	.01	.002	.001
2.	19.424	49.427	99.427	499.417	999.376
3.	8.716	16.695	26.923	80.264	128.036
4.	5.873	9.817	14.246	32.943	46.939
5.	4.636	7.156	9.769	19.503	26.045
6.	3.956	5.797	7.604	13.803	17.686
7.	3.529	4.985	6.359	10.801	13.435
8.	3.237	4.450	5.559	8.990	10.943
9.	3.026	4.071	5.005	7.796	9.335
10.	2.865	3.790	4.601	6.955	8.220
11.	2.739	3.573	4.293	6.335	7.409
12.	2.637	3.402	4.052	5.860	6.794
13.	2.554	3.262	3.857	5.486	6.314
14.	2.484	3.146	3.697	5.184	5.930
15.	2.424	3.049	3.564	4.935	5.615
16.	2.373	2.966	3.451	4.727	5.353
17.	2.329	2.894	3.353	4.550	5.132
18.	2.290	2.832	3.269	4.399	4.943
19.	2.256	2.777	3.195	4.267	4.780
20.	2.225	2.728	3.130	4.152	4.637
21.	2.198	2.685	3.072	4.050	4.512
22.	2.173	2.646	3.019	3.959	4.401
23.	2.150	2.610	2.973	3.878	4.301
24.	2.130	2.578	2.930	3.806	4.212
25.	2.111	2.549	2.892	3.740	4.132
26.	2.094	2.523	2.857	3.680	4.059
27.	2.078	2.498	2.824	3.625	3.993
28.	2.064	2.476	2.795	3.575	3.932
29.	2.050	2.455	2.767	3.529	3.876
30.	2.037	2.435	2.742	3.486	3.825
31.	2.026	2.417	2.718	3.447	3.777
32.	2.015	2.400	2.696	3.410	3.733
33.	2.004	2.385	2.676	3.376	3.692
34.	1.995	2.370	2.657	3.345	3.654
35.	1.986	2.356	2.639	3.315	3.618
36.	1.977	2.343	2.622	3.287	3.585
37.	1.969	2.331	2.606	3.261	3.554
38.	1.962	2.319	2.591	3.237	3.524
39.	1.954	2.309	2.577	3.213	3.497
40.	1.948	2.298	2.563	3.192	3.471
50.	1.895	2.219	2.461	3.026	3.273
60.	1.860	2.167	2.394	2.920	3.147
70.	1.836	2.130	2.348	2.846	3.060
80.	1.817	2.103	2.313	2.791	2.996
90.	1.803	2.082	2.287	2.750	2.947
100.	1.792	2.066	2.265	2.717	2.908

Degrees of Freedom for the Numerator = 15

df for the Denomina-tor	Probability Level				
	.05	.02	.01	.002	.001
2.	19.429	49.432	99.434	499.432	999.401
3.	8.701	16.658	26.853	79.966	127.675
4.	5.858	9.780	14.194	32.801	46.776
5.	4.619	7.124	9.722	19.409	25.907
6.	3.938	5.764	7.559	13.713	17.561
7.	3.511	4.954	6.314	10.714	13.325
8.	3.218	4.417	5.515	8.909	10.843
9.	3.006	4.039	4.962	7.718	9.239
10.	2.845	3.758	4.558	6.881	8.129
11.	2.719	3.541	4.251	6.263	7.322
12.	2.617	3.369	4.010	5.789	6.710
13.	2.533	3.230	3.815	5.417	6.231
14.	2.463	3.114	3.656	5.116	5.848
15.	2.403	3.017	3.522	4.868	5.535
16.	2.352	2.934	3.409	4.660	5.274
17.	2.308	2.862	3.312	4.484	5.054
18.	2.269	2.799	3.227	4.333	4.866
19.	2.234	2.744	3.153	4.202	4.704
20.	2.203	2.695	3.088	4.087	4.562
21.	2.176	2.652	3.030	3.986	4.437
22.	2.151	2.613	2.978	3.895	4.326
23.	2.128	2.578	2.931	3.815	4.227
24.	2.108	2.545	2.889	3.742	4.139
25.	2.089	2.516	2.850	3.676	4.059
26.	2.072	2.489	2.815	3.617	3.986
27.	2.056	2.465	2.783	3.562	3.920
28.	2.041	2.442	2.753	3.512	3.859
29.	2.027	2.421	2.726	3.466	3.804
30.	2.015	2.402	2.700	3.424	3.753
31.	2.003	2.384	2.677	3.385	3.706
32.	1.992	2.367	2.655	3.348	3.662
33.	1.982	2.351	2.634	3.314	3.621
34.	1.972	2.337	2.615	3.283	3.583
35.	1.963	2.323	2.597	3.253	3.548
36.	1.954	2.310	2.580	3.226	3.514
37.	1.946	2.297	2.564	3.199	3.483
38.	1.939	2.286	2.549	3.175	3.454
39.	1.931	2.275	2.535	3.152	3.426
40.	1.924	2.264	2.522	3.130	3.400
50.	1.871	2.185	2.419	2.965	3.204
60.	1.836	2.133	2.352	2.859	3.078
70.	1.812	2.096	2.306	2.785	2.991
80.	1.793	2.069	2.271	2.731	2.927
90.	1.779	2.048	2.244	2.689	2.879
100.	1.768	2.031	2.223	2.656	2.840

Degrees of Freedom for the Numerator = 16

df for the Denomina-tor	Probability Level				
	.05	.02	.01	.002	.001
2.	19.434	49.437	99.438	499.439	999.410
3.	8.694	16.634	26.849	79.865	127.149
4.	5.844	9.755	14.154	32.683	46.628
5.	4.604	7.096	9.680	19.314	25.793
6.	3.923	5.736	7.518	13.632	17.453
7.	3.494	4.925	6.275	10.639	13.226
8.	3.202	4.390	5.477	8.837	10.751
9.	2.989	4.011	4.924	7.650	9.153
10.	2.828	3.730	4.520	6.815	8.048
11.	2.701	3.513	4.213	6.199	7.243
12.	2.599	3.341	3.972	5.728	6.634
13.	2.515	3.202	3.778	5.356	6.158
14.	2.445	3.086	3.619	5.055	5.776
15.	2.385	2.988	3.485	4.809	5.464
16.	2.334	2.905	3.372	4.602	5.205
17.	2.289	2.833	3.275	4.426	4.985
18.	2.250	2.770	3.190	4.275	4.798
19.	2.215	2.715	3.117	4.145	4.636
20.	2.184	2.667	3.051	4.030	4.495
21.	2.156	2.623	2.993	3.929	4.371
22.	2.131	2.584	2.941	3.839	4.260
23.	2.109	2.548	2.894	3.758	4.162
24.	2.088	2.516	2.852	3.686	4.074
25.	2.069	2.487	2.813	3.620	3.994
26.	2.052	2.460	2.778	3.561	3.922
27.	2.036	2.436	2.746	3.506	3.856
28.	2.021	2.413	2.716	3.457	3.795
29.	2.007	2.392	2.689	3.411	3.740
30.	1.995	2.372	2.663	3.369	3.689
31.	1.983	2.354	2.640	3.329	3.642
32.	1.972	2.337	2.618	3.293	3.598
33.	1.961	2.322	2.597	3.259	3.558
34.	1.952	2.307	2.578	3.228	3.520
35.	1.942	2.293	2.560	3.198	3.484
36.	1.934	2.280	2.543	3.171	3.451
37.	1.926	2.268	2.527	3.145	3.420
38.	1.918	2.256	2.512	3.120	3.391
39.	1.911	2.245	2.498	3.097	3.364
40.	1.904	2.235	2.484	3.076	3.338
50.	1.850	2.155	2.382	2.911	3.142
60.	1.815	2.102	2.315	2.805	3.017
70.	1.790	2.065	2.268	2.731	2.930
80.	1.772	2.038	2.233	2.677	2.867
90.	1.757	2.017	2.206	2.636	2.818
100.	1.746	2.000	2.185	2.603	2.779

Degrees of Freedom for the Numerator = 17

df for the Denomina-tor	Probability Level				
	.05	.02	.01	.002	.001
2.	19.437	49.440	99.442	499.442	999.416
3.	8.682	16.597	26.813	79.859	127.615
4.	5.832	9.729	14.116	32.609	46.422
5.	4.590	7.070	9.644	19.225	25.666
6.	3.908	5.711	7.484	13.560	17.351
7.	3.480	4.900	6.241	10.574	13.139
8.	3.187	4.364	5.443	8.776	10.673
9.	2.974	3.986	4.890	7.589	9.078
10.	2.812	3.705	4.487	6.757	7.978
11.	2.685	3.488	4.180	6.143	7.175
12.	2.583	3.316	3.939	5.672	6.567
13.	2.499	3.176	3.745	5.301	6.092
14.	2.428	3.060	3.586	5.002	5.712
15.	2.368	2.963	3.452	4.756	5.401
16.	2.317	2.879	3.339	4.549	5.143
17.	2.272	2.807	3.242	4.374	4.924
18.	2.233	2.745	3.158	4.224	4.738
19.	2.198	2.689	3.084	4.093	4.576
20.	2.167	2.641	3.018	3.979	4.435
21.	2.139	2.597	2.960	3.878	4.311
22.	2.114	2.558	2.908	3.788	4.202
23.	2.091	2.522	2.861	3.708	4.103
24.	2.070	2.490	2.819	3.636	4.015
25.	2.051	2.461	2.780	3.570	3.936
26.	2.034	2.434	2.745	3.511	3.864
27.	2.018	2.409	2.713	3.457	3.798
28.	2.003	2.386	2.683	3.407	3.738
29.	1.989	2.365	2.655	3.361	3.683
30.	1.977	2.346	2.630	3.319	3.632
31.	1.965	2.328	2.607	3.280	3.585
32.	1.953	2.311	2.584	3.244	3.542
33.	1.943	2.295	2.564	3.210	3.501
34.	1.933	2.280	2.545	3.179	3.463
35.	1.924	2.266	2.527	3.149	3.428
36.	1.915	2.253	2.510	3.122	3.395
37.	1.907	2.241	2.494	3.096	3.364
38.	1.899	2.229	2.479	3.071	3.335
39.	1.892	2.218	2.465	3.048	3.308
40.	1.885	2.208	2.451	3.027	3.282
50.	1.831	2.127	2.348	2.862	3.086
60.	1.796	2.075	2.281	2.756	2.962
70.	1.771	2.038	2.234	2.683	2.875
80.	1.752	2.010	2.199	2.629	2.812
90.	1.737	1.989	2.173	2.587	2.763
100.	1.726	1.972	2.151	2.554	2.725

Degrees of Freedom for the Numerator = 18

df for the Denomina-tor	Probability Level				
	.05	.02	.01	.002	.001
2.	19.441	49.444	99.445	499.447	999.420
3.	8.674	16.599	26.770	79.853	126.107
4.	5.822	9.709	14.077	32.542	46.381
5.	4.579	7.046	9.608	19.140	25.562
6.	3.896	5.689	7.451	13.488	17.263
7.	3.467	4.877	6.209	10.514	13.064
8.	3.173	4.342	5.412	8.719	10.599
9.	2.960	3.963	4.860	7.536	9.013
10.	2.798	3.682	4.457	6.705	7.913
11.	2.671	3.465	4.150	6.092	7.114
12.	2.568	3.294	3.909	5.623	6.507
13.	2.484	3.153	3.716	5.253	6.034
14.	2.413	3.037	3.556	4.954	5.655
15.	2.353	2.940	3.423	4.708	5.345
16.	2.302	2.856	3.309	4.502	5.087
17.	2.257	2.784	3.213	4.327	4.869
18.	2.217	2.722	3.128	4.178	4.683
19.	2.182	2.666	3.054	4.047	4.522
20.	2.151	2.617	2.989	3.933	4.382
21.	2.123	2.574	2.931	3.832	4.258
22.	2.098	2.534	2.879	3.743	4.149
23.	2.075	2.499	2.832	3.663	4.051
24.	2.054	2.466	2.789	3.591	3.963
25.	2.035	2.437	2.751	3.526	3.884
26.	2.018	2.410	2.715	3.466	3.812
27.	2.002	2.385	2.683	3.412	3.747
28.	1.987	2.363	2.653	3.363	3.686
29.	1.973	2.342	2.626	3.317	3.632
30.	1.960	2.322	2.600	3.275	3.581
31.	1.948	2.304	2.577	3.236	3.534
32.	1.937	2.287	2.555	3.200	3.491
33.	1.926	2.271	2.534	3.166	3.450
34.	1.917	2.256	2.515	3.135	3.413
35.	1.907	2.242	2.497	3.105	3.377
36.	1.899	2.229	2.480	3.078	3.345
37.	1.890	2.216	2.464	3.052	3.314
38.	1.883	2.205	2.449	3.027	3.285
39.	1.875	2.194	2.435	3.004	3.257
40.	1.868	2.183	2.421	2.983	3.232
50.	1.814	2.103	2.318	2.818	3.037
60.	1.778	2.050	2.251	2.713	2.912
70.	1.753	2.013	2.204	2.639	2.826
80.	1.734	1.985	2.169	2.585	2.763
90.	1.720	1.964	2.142	2.544	2.714
100.	1.708	1.947	2.120	2.511	2.676

Degrees of Freedom for the Numerator = 19

df for the Denomina- tor	Probability Level				
	.05	.02	.01	.002	.001
2.	19.443	49.446	99.446	499.440	999.405
3.	8.668	16.573	26.685	79.748	126.809
4.	5.810	9.690	14.050	32.445	46.166
5.	4.568	7.028	9.578	19.082	25.458
6.	3.884	5.670	7.422	13.431	17.186
7.	3.455	4.857	6.181	10.456	12.997
8.	3.161	4.321	5.384	8.669	10.536
9.	2.948	3.943	4.832	7.487	8.952
10.	2.785	3.662	4.430	6.659	7.855
11.	2.658	3.445	4.124	6.047	7.058
12.	2.555	3.273	3.883	5.578	6.453
13.	2.471	3.133	3.689	5.208	5.982
14.	2.400	3.017	3.530	4.911	5.603
15.	2.340	2.919	3.396	4.665	5.294
16.	2.288	2.836	3.283	4.460	5.037
17.	2.243	2.764	3.186	4.285	4.820
18.	2.203	2.701	3.101	4.136	4.634
19.	2.168	2.645	3.027	4.006	4.474
20.	2.137	2.596	2.962	3.892	4.334
21.	2.109	2.552	2.904	3.791	4.210
22.	2.084	2.513	2.852	3.702	4.101
23.	2.061	2.477	2.805	3.622	4.003
24.	2.040	2.445	2.762	3.550	3.916
25.	2.021	2.416	2.724	3.485	3.837
26.	2.003	2.389	2.689	3.426	3.765
27.	1.987	2.364	2.656	3.372	3.700
28.	1.972	2.341	2.626	3.322	3.640
29.	1.958	2.320	2.599	3.277	3.585
30.	1.945	2.300	2.573	3.235	3.535
31.	1.933	2.282	2.550	3.196	3.488
32.	1.922	2.265	2.527	3.160	3.445
33.	1.911	2.249	2.507	3.126	3.404
34.	1.901	2.234	2.488	3.094	3.367
35.	1.892	2.220	2.470	3.065	3.332
36.	1.883	2.207	2.453	3.038	3.299
37.	1.875	2.195	2.437	3.012	3.268
38.	1.867	2.183	2.421	2.987	3.239
39.	1.860	2.172	2.407	2.965	3.212
40.	1.853	2.161	2.394	2.943	3.186
50.	1.798	2.080	2.290	2.779	2.992
60.	1.763	2.027	2.223	2.673	2.867
70.	1.737	1.990	2.176	2.600	2.781
80.	1.718	1.962	2.141	2.546	2.718
90.	1.703	1.941	2.114	2.504	2.670
100.	1.691	1.924	2.092	2.471	2.632

Degrees of Freedom for the Numerator = 20

df for the Denomina-tor	Probability Level				
	.05	.02	.01	.002	.001
2.	19.446	49.449	99.449	499.445	999.410
3.	8.663	16.554	26.672	79.448	126.694
4.	5.803	9.666	14.024	32.364	46.034
5.	4.558	7.011	9.552	19.014	25.410
6.	3.874	5.652	7.397	13.377	17.122
7.	3.445	4.839	6.156	10.411	12.928
8.	3.150	4.303	5.360	8.622	10.480
9.	2.936	3.925	4.808	7.445	8.899
10.	2.774	3.644	4.405	6.617	7.803
11.	2.646	3.427	4.099	6.005	7.007
12.	2.544	3.254	3.858	5.538	6.405
13.	2.459	3.114	3.664	5.169	5.933
14.	2.388	2.998	3.505	4.872	5.556
15.	2.327	2.900	3.372	4.627	5.248
16.	2.276	2.817	3.259	4.422	4.992
17.	2.230	2.744	3.161	4.247	4.775
18.	2.191	2.682	3.077	4.098	4.590
19.	2.155	2.626	3.003	3.968	4.429
20.	2.124	2.577	2.938	3.855	4.290
21.	2.096	2.533	2.880	3.754	4.167
22.	2.071	2.494	2.827	3.665	4.058
23.	2.048	2.458	2.781	3.585	3.960
24.	2.027	2.426	2.738	3.513	3.873
25.	2.007	2.396	2.699	3.448	3.794
26.	1.990	2.369	2.664	3.389	3.723
27.	1.974	2.344	2.632	3.335	3.658
28.	1.959	2.321	2.602	3.286	3.598
29.	1.945	2.300	2.574	3.240	3.543
30.	1.932	2.281	2.549	3.198	3.493
31.	1.920	2.262	2.525	3.159	3.446
32.	1.908	2.245	2.503	3.123	3.403
33.	1.898	2.229	2.482	3.090	3.363
34.	1.888	2.214	2.463	3.058	3.325
35.	1.878	2.200	2.445	3.029	3.290
36.	1.870	2.187	2.428	3.001	3.258
37.	1.861	2.174	2.412	2.976	3.227
38.	1.853	2.163	2.397	2.951	3.198
39.	1.846	2.152	2.382	2.928	3.171
40.	1.839	2.141	2.369	2.907	3.145
50.	1.784	2.060	2.265	2.742	2.951
60.	1.748	2.007	2.198	2.637	2.827
70.	1.722	1.969	2.150	2.564	2.741
80.	1.703	1.941	2.115	2.509	2.677
90.	1.688	1.920	2.088	2.468	2.629
100.	1.676	1.903	2.067	2.435	2.591

Degrees of Freedom for the Numerator = 25

df for the Denomina-tor	Probability Level				
	.05	.02	.01	.002	.001
2.	19.456	49.458	99.459	499.453	999.417
3.	8.633	16.489	26.584	78.918	125.709
4.	5.769	9.599	13.905	32.054	45.730
5.	4.521	6.941	9.448	18.782	25.079
6.	3.835	5.580	7.295	13.175	16.847
7.	3.404	4.769	6.057	10.221	12.693
8.	3.108	4.234	5.263	8.446	10.258
9.	2.893	3.854	4.713	7.276	8.688
10.	2.730	3.573	4.311	6.453	7.603
11.	2.601	3.355	4.005	5.847	6.815
12.	2.498	3.183	3.765	5.382	6.217
13.	2.412	3.042	3.571	5.016	5.751
14.	2.341	2.926	3.412	4.720	5.377
15.	2.280	2.827	3.278	4.477	5.071
16.	2.227	2.743	3.165	4.273	4.817
17.	2.182	2.671	3.068	4.100	4.602
18.	2.141	2.608	2.983	3.952	4.418
19.	2.106	2.552	2.909	3.823	4.259
20.	2.074	2.502	2.843	3.709	4.121
21.	2.045	2.458	2.785	3.610	3.999
22.	2.020	2.418	2.733	3.521	3.890
23.	1.996	2.382	2.686	3.442	3.794
24.	1.975	2.350	2.643	3.370	3.707
25.	1.955	2.320	2.604	3.305	3.629
26.	1.938	2.293	2.569	3.246	3.558
27.	1.921	2.268	2.536	3.192	3.493
28.	1.906	2.244	2.506	3.143	3.434
29.	1.891	2.223	2.478	3.098	3.380
30.	1.878	2.203	2.453	3.056	3.329
31.	1.866	2.185	2.429	3.017	3.283
32.	1.854	2.167	2.406	2.981	3.240
33.	1.844	2.151	2.386	2.948	3.200
34.	1.833	2.136	2.366	2.917	3.163
35.	1.824	2.122	2.348	2.887	3.128
36.	1.815	2.108	2.331	2.860	3.096
37.	1.806	2.096	2.315	2.834	3.065
38.	1.798	2.084	2.299	2.810	3.036
39.	1.791	2.073	2.285	2.787	3.009
40.	1.783	2.062	2.271	2.765	2.984
50.	1.727	1.979	2.167	2.601	2.790
60.	1.690	1.925	2.098	2.495	2.666
70.	1.664	1.887	2.050	2.422	2.581
80.	1.644	1.858	2.015	2.368	2.518
90.	1.629	1.836	1.987	2.326	2.469
100.	1.616	1.819	1.965	2.293	2.431

Degrees of Freedom for the Numerator = 30

df for the Denominator	Probability Level				
	.05	.02	.01	.002	.001
2.	19.462	49.464	99.464	499.449	999.403
3.	8.617	16.448	26.504	78.781	125.445
4.	5.745	9.549	13.836	31.933	45.497
5.	4.496	6.892	9.377	18.649	24.857
6.	3.808	5.535	7.228	13.046	16.680
7.	3.376	4.723	5.992	10.095	12.526
8.	3.080	4.185	5.199	8.328	10.108
9.	2.864	3.807	4.648	7.163	8.546
10.	2.700	3.525	4.247	6.342	7.470
11.	2.570	3.307	3.941	5.739	6.683
12.	2.466	3.134	3.701	5.276	6.090
13.	2.380	2.993	3.507	4.912	5.626
14.	2.308	2.876	3.347	4.617	5.254
15.	2.247	2.778	3.214	4.375	4.950
16.	2.194	2.693	3.101	4.172	4.697
17.	2.148	2.620	3.003	4.000	4.484
18.	2.107	2.557	2.919	3.851	4.301
19.	2.071	2.501	2.844	3.723	4.143
20.	2.039	2.451	2.779	3.610	4.005
21.	2.010	2.406	2.720	3.511	3.884
22.	1.984	2.366	2.668	3.422	3.776
23.	1.961	2.330	2.620	3.343	3.680
24.	1.939	2.297	2.577	3.271	3.593
25.	1.919	2.267	2.538	3.207	3.515
26.	1.901	2.240	2.503	3.148	3.445
27.	1.884	2.214	2.470	3.094	3.380
28.	1.869	2.191	2.440	3.045	3.321
29.	1.854	2.169	2.412	3.000	3.267
30.	1.841	2.149	2.386	2.958	3.217
31.	1.828	2.131	2.362	2.919	3.171
32.	1.817	2.113	2.340	2.883	3.128
33.	1.806	2.097	2.319	2.850	3.088
34.	1.795	2.082	2.299	2.818	3.051
35.	1.786	2.067	2.281	2.789	3.016
36.	1.776	2.054	2.263	2.762	2.984
37.	1.768	2.041	2.247	2.736	2.953
38.	1.760	2.029	2.232	2.712	2.925
39.	1.752	2.017	2.217	2.689	2.898
40.	1.744	2.006	2.203	2.667	2.872
50.	1.687	1.923	2.098	2.503	2.679
60.	1.649	1.868	2.028	2.397	2.555
70.	1.622	1.829	1.980	2.323	2.469
80.	1.602	1.800	1.944	2.268	2.406
90.	1.586	1.777	1.916	2.226	2.357
100.	1.573	1.759	1.893	2.193	2.319

Appendix H

Table of Critical Values for the t-Test (one-tailed)*

Degrees of Freedom	Probability Level				
	.05	.02	.01	.002	.001
2.	2.920	4.849	6.965	15.764	22.327
3.	2.353	3.482	4.541	8.053	10.215
4.	2.132	2.999	3.747	5.951	7.173
5.	2.015	2.757	3.365	5.030	5.893
6.	1.943	2.612	3.143	4.524	5.208
7.	1.895	2.517	2.998	4.207	4.785
8.	1.860	2.449	2.896	3.991	4.501
9.	1.833	2.398	2.821	3.835	4.297
10.	1.812	2.359	2.764	3.716	4.144
11.	1.796	2.328	2.718	3.624	4.025
12.	1.782	2.303	2.681	3.550	3.930
13.	1.771	2.282	2.650	3.489	3.852
14.	1.761	2.264	2.624	3.438	3.787
15.	1.753	2.249	2.602	3.395	3.733
16.	1.746	2.235	2.583	3.358	3.686
17.	1.740	2.224	2.567	3.326	3.646
18.	1.734	2.214	2.552	3.298	3.610
19.	1.729	2.205	2.539	3.273	3.579
20.	1.725	2.197	2.528	3.251	3.552
21.	1.721	2.189	2.518	3.231	3.527
22.	1.717	2.183	2.508	3.214	3.505
23.	1.714	2.177	2.500	3.198	3.485
24.	1.711	2.172	2.492	3.183	3.467
25.	1.708	2.167	2.485	3.170	3.450
26.	1.706	2.162	2.479	3.158	3.435
27.	1.703	2.158	2.473	3.147	3.421
28.	1.701	2.154	2.467	3.136	3.408
29.	1.699	2.150	2.462	3.127	3.396
30.	1.697	2.147	2.457	3.118	3.385

* The values for this table were generated by computer, using a FORTRAN (MDSTI) program.

Appendix I

Table of Critical Values for the Chi Square*

Degrees of Freedom	Probability Level				
	.05	.02	.01	.002	.001
2.	5.99	7.82	9.22	12.43	13.69
3.	7.82	9.84	11.32	14.75	16.29
4.	9.49	11.68	13.28	16.83	18.43
5.	11.07	13.40	15.09	18.92	20.75
6.	12.60	15.04	16.81	20.78	22.68
7.	14.07	16.63	18.47	22.56	24.53
8.	15.51	18.18	20.08	24.29	26.32
9.	16.93	19.69	21.65	26.18	28.06
10.	18.31	21.17	23.19	27.84	29.76
11.	19.68	22.63	24.75	29.47	31.43
12.	21.03	24.07	26.25	31.07	33.07
13.	22.37	25.48	27.72	32.64	34.68
14	23.69	26.89	29.17	34.20	36.27
15	25.00	28.27	30.61	35.73	37.84
16.	26.30	29.65	32.03	37.24	39.39
17	27.59	31.01	33.44	38.74	40.93
18.	28.88	32.36	34.83	40.23	42.44
19.	30.15	33.71	36.22	41.70	43.95
20.	31.42	35.03	37.59	43.16	45.44
21.	32.68	36.36	38.96	44.61	46.92
22.	33.93	37.67	40.31	46.05	48.39
23.	35.18	38.99	41.66	47.47	49.84
24.	36.42	40.28	43.00	48.89	51.29
25.	37.66	41.58	44.34	50.30	52.73
26.	38.89	42.88	45.66	51.71	54.16
27.	40.12	44.16	46.99	53.10	55.58
28.	41.34	45.44	48.30	54.49	57.00
29.	42.56	46.71	49.61	55.87	58.40
30.	43.78	47.98	50.91	57.24	59.81

* The values for this table were generated by computer, using a FORTRAN (MDCHI) program.

References

Adams, M. Vocal characteristics of normal speakers and stutterers during choral reading. *J. Speech Hearing Res.*, 23, 457–470, 1980.

Adams, M., and Ramig, P., Vocal characteristics of normal speakers and stutterers during choral reading. *J. Speech Hearing Res.*, 23, 457–469, 1980.

Arnold, K., and Emanuel, F., Spectral noise levels and roughness severity ratings for vowels produced by male children. *J. Speech Hearing Res.*, 22, 613–626, 1979.

Austin, G., Knowledge of Selected concepts obtained by an adolescent deaf population. *Amer. Ann. Deaf*, 120, 360–370, 1975.

Behnke, C., and Lankford, J., The LOT test and school-age children. *J. Speech Hearing Dis.* 41, 498–502, 1976.

Bloodstein, O., and Gantwerk, B., Grammatical function in relation to stuttering in young children. *J. Speech Hearing Res.*, 10, 786–789, 1967.

Bond, Z., and Wilson, H., Acquisition of the voicing contrast by language-delayed and normal-speaking children. *J. Speech Hearing Res.*, 23, 152–161, 1980.

Bountress, N., Comprehension of pronominal reference by speakers of Black English. *J. Speech Hearing Res.*, 21, 96–102, 1978.

Brasel, K., and Quigley, S., Influence of certain language and communication environments in early childhood on the development of language in deaf individuals. *J. Speech Hearing Res.*, 20, 95–107, 1977.

Brookshire, R., and Nicholas, L., Verification of active and passive sentences by aphasic and nonaphasic subjects. *J. Speech Hearing Res.*, 23, 878–893, 1980.

Bruning, J., and Kintz, B., *Computational Handbook of Statistics*. Glenview, Ill., Scott Foresman, 1977.

Bruns, J., Gram, J., and Rogers, G., Impedance and otoscopy screening of multiply handicapped children. *Lang. Speech Hearing Serv. School*, 10, 54–58, 1979.

Campbell, D., and Stanley, J., *Experimental and Quasi-Experimental Designs for Research*. Chicago: Rand McNally, 1963.

Cecconi, C., Hood, S., and Tucker, R., Influence of reading level difficulty on the disfluencies of normal children. *J. Speech Hearing Res.*, 20, 475–478, 1977.

Chaiklin, J., and Ventry, I., Spondee threshold measurement: A comparison of 2 and 5 dB methods. *J. Speech Hearing Dis.*, 29, 47–59, 1964.

Chapman, R., and Kohn, L., Comprehension strategies in two and three year olds: animate agents or probable events. *J. Speech Hearing Res.*, 21, 746–761, 1978.

Chuang, C., and Wang, W., Use of optical distance sensing to track tongue motion. *J. Speech Hearing Dis.*, 21, 482–496, 1978.

Cook, J., Palaski, D., Hanson, W., A vocal hygiene program for school-age children. *Lang. Speech Hearing Serv. Schools*, 10, 21–26, 1979.

Costello, J., and Schoen, J., The effectiveness of paraprofessionals and speech clinicians as agents of articulation intervention using programmed instruction. *Lang. Speech Hearing Serv. Schools*, 9, 118–128, 1978.

Cottrell, A., Montague, J., Farb, J., and Throve, J., An operant procedure for improving vocabulary definition performances in developmentally delayed children. *J. Speech Hearing Dis.*, 45, 90–102, 1980.

Daly, D., and Kimbarow, M., Stuttering as operant behavior: Effects of the verbal stimuli wrong, right and three of the disfluency rates of school-age stutterers and nonstutterers. *J. Speech Hearing Res.*, 21, 589–597, 1978.

Davis, H., *Hearing and Deafness*. New York: Holt, Rinehart, Winston, 1947.

DeHirsch, K., Jansky, J., and Langford, W., The oral language performance of premature children and controls. *J. Speech Hearing Dis.* 29, 60–69, 1964.

Dice, G., and Shearer, W., Clinician's accuracy in detecting vocal nodules, *Lang. Speech Hearing Serv. Schools*, 4, 142–144, 1973.

Downie, N., and Heath, R., *Basic Statistical Methods*. New York: Harper & Row, 1959.

DuBois, E., and Bernthal, J., A comparison of three methods for obtaining articulation responses. *J. Speech Hearing Dis.*, 43, 295–305, 1978.

Dworkin, J., Protrusive Lingual force and lingual diadochokinetic rates: A comparative analysis between normal and lisping speakers. *Lang. Speech Hearing Serv. Schools*, 9, 8–16, 1978.

Eilers, R., and Oller, K., A comparative study of speech perception in young severely retarded children and normally developing infants., *J. Speech Hearing Res.*, 23, 419–428, 1980.

Ferguson, G., *Statistical Analysis in Psychology and Education*, New York: McGraw-Hill, 1971.

Fletcher, S., McCutcheon, M., and Wolf, M., Dynamic palatometry. *J. Speech Hearing Res.*, 18, 812–819, 1975.

Folger, M., and Leonard, L., Language and Sensorimotor development during the early period of referential speech. *J. Speech Hearing Res.*, 21, 519–527, 1978.

Franks, J., Cooper, W., and McFall, R., Filter effects of earmold venting: Comparison of electroacoustic and psychoacoustic methods of evaluation. *J. Am. Audiological Soc.*, 3, 6–9, 1977.

Franks, J., and Daniloff, R., A review of the audiological implications of testing vowel perception. *J. Auditory Res.*, 13, 355–368, 1973.

Freeman, B., and Beasley, D., Discrimination of Time-altered sentential approximations and monosyllables by children with reading problems. *J. Speech Hearing Res.* 506, 1978.

Garber, S., and Moller, K., The effects of feedback filtering on nasalization in normal and hypernasal speakers. *J Speech Hearing Res.*, 22, 231–333, 1979.

Giolas, T., Owens, E., Lamb, S., and Schubert, E., Hearing performance inventory. *J. Speech Hearing Dis.*, 44, 169–195, 1979.

Glaser, E., McWilliams, B., Skolnick, M., Response to Bowman and Shanks. *J. Speech Hearing Dis.*, 44, 557–558, 1979.

Griggs, S., and Still, A., An analysis of individual differences in words stuttered. *J. Speech Hearing Res.*, 22, 572–580, 1979.

Guilford, J., *Fundamental Statistics in Psychology and Education*, New York: McGraw-Hill, 1956.

Harford, E., and Barry, J., A rehabilitative approach to the unilateral hearing impairment: the contralateral routing of signals (CROS). *J. Speech Hearing Dis.*, 30, 121–138, 1965.

Haskell, J., and Baker, R., Self-perception of speaking pitch levels. *J. Speech Hearing Dis.*, 43, 3–8, 1978.

Hays, W., *Statistics for the Social Sciences*, (2nd Ed.), Holt, Rinehart, Winston, 1973.

Haynes, W., and Oratio, A., a study of clients' perceptions of therapeutic effectiveness. *J. Speech Hearing Dis.*, 43, 21–23, 1978.

Healey, C., Mallard, A., and Adams, M., Factors contributing to the reduction of stuttering during singing. *J. Speech Hearing Res.*, 19, 475–480, 1976.

Hixon T., Mead, J., and Goldman, M., Dynamics of chest wall during speech production: Function of the thorax, rib cage, diaphragm, and abdomen. *J. Speech Hearing Res.*, 19, 297–356, 1976.

Hollien, H., Vocal fold thickness and fundamental frequency of phonation. *J. Speech Hearing Res.*, 5, 237–243, 1962.

Horovitz, L., Johnson, S., Pearlman, R., Schaffer, E., and Hedin, A., Stapedial reflex and anxiety in fluent and disfluent speakers. *J. Speech Hearing Res.*, 764–767, 1978.

Hudgens, J. and Culliman, W., Effects of sentence structure on sentence elicited imitation responses. *J. Speech Hearing Res.* 21, 808–819, 1978.

Huggins, A., Better spectrograms from children's speech. *J. Speech Hearing Res.*, 23, 19–27, 1980.

Iglesias, A., Kuehn, D., Morris, H., Simultaneous assessment of pharyngeal wall and velar displacement for selected speech sounds. *J. Speech Hearing Res.*, 23, 429–446, 1980.

Jackson, P., Montgomery, A., and Binnie, C., Perceptual dimensions underlying vowel lipreading performance. *J. Speech Hearing Res.*, 19, 796–812, 1976.

Jerger, J., Viewpoint. *J. Speech Hearing Res.*, 6, 301, 1963.

Johnson, W., People in Quandaries: The Semantics of Personal Adjustment. New York: Harper Brothers, 1946.

Kirk, R., *Experimental Design: Procedures for the Behavioral Sciences*. Belmont, Cal.: Brooks-Cole, 1968.

Kresheck, J., and Socolofsky, G., Imitative and spontaneous articulatory assessment of four-year-old children. *J. Speech Hearing Res.*, 15, 729–733, 1972.

Lankford, J., and Behnke, C., Bacteriology of and cleaning methods for stock earmolds. *J. Speech Hearing Res.*, 16, 325–329, 1973.

Laughlin, S., Naeser, M., and Gordon, W., Effects of three syllable durations using the melodic intonation therapy technique. *J. Speech Hearing Res.*, 22, 311–333, 1979.

Lindquist, E., *Design and Analysis of Experiments in Psychology and Education*. New York: Houghton Mifflin, 1953.

Logemann, J., and Fisher, H., Boshes, B., and Blousky, R., Frequency and concurrence of vocal tract dysfunctions in the speech of a large sample of Parkinson patients. *J. Speech Hearing Dis.*, 43, 47–57, 1978.

Love, R., Hagerman, E., and Taimi, E., Speech performance dysphasia and oral reflexes in cerebral palsy. *J. Speech Hearing Dis.*, 45, 59–75, 1980.

Matheny, N., and Panagos, J., Comparing the effects of articulation and syntax programs on syntax and articulation improvement. *Lang. Speech Hearing Serv. Schools*, 9, 57–61, 1978.

Mallory, Y. and Chapman, D., Sequential Features of black child language. *Lang Speech Hearing Serv. Schools*, 4, 204–209, 1978.

Menon, K., and Shearer, W., Hyoid position during repeated syllables. *J. Speech Hearing Res.*, 14, 858–864, 1971.

Mills, R., Knox, A., Juola, J., and Salmon, S., Cognitive loci of impairments in picture naming by aphasic subjects. *J. Speech Hearing Res.*, 22, 73–87, 1979.

Monroe, D., and Martin, F., Effects of sophistication on four tests for nonorganic hearing loss. *J. Speech Hearing Dis.* 42, 528–534, 1977.

Monsen, R. Second formant transitions of selected consonant-vowel combinations in the speech of deaf and normal-hearing children. *J. Speech Hearing Dis.*, 19, 277–289, 1976.

Myers, J., *Fundmentals of Experimental Design.* 2nd ed., New York: Allyn and Bacon, 1972.

Oller, D., Payne, S., and Gavin, W. Tactual speech perception by minimally trained deaf subjects. *J. Speech Hearing Res.*, 23, 757–768, 1980.

Orchik, D., Drygier, K., and Cutts, B., A comparison for the NU-6 and W-22 speech discrimination tests for assessing sensorineural hearing loss. *J. Speech Hearing Dis.*, 44, 522–527, 1979.

Panagos, J., and King, R., Self and mutual speech comprehension by deviant- and normal-speaking children. *J. Speech Hearing Res.*, 18, 653–662, 1975.

Panagos, J., Quine, M., and Klick, R., Syntactic and phonological influences on children's articulation. *J. Speech Hearing Res.* 22, 841–848, 1979.

Penner, J., Two-tone foreward masking patterns and tinnitus. *J. Speech Hearing Res.*, 23, 779–786, 1980.

Platt, L., Andrews, G., Young, M., and Quinn, P., Dysarthria of adult cerebral palsy: I. Intelligibility and Articulatory impairment. *J. Speech Hearing Res.*, 23, 28–40, 1980.

Prosek, R., Montgomery, A., Walden, B., and Schwartz, D., EMG Biofeedback in the treatment of hyperfunctional voice disorders, *J. Speech Hearing Res.*, 43, 282–294, 1978.

Punch, J., and Beck, E., Low-frequency response of hearing aids and judgements of aided speech quality. *J. Speech Hearing Dis.*, 45, 325–335, 1980.

Ratusnik, D., Klee, T., and Ratusnik, C., Northwestern syntax screening test: a short form. *J. Speech Hearing Dis.*, 45, 200–208, 1980.

Reed, C., and Lingwell, J., Conditioned stimulus effects on stuttering and GSRs. *J. Speech Hearing Res.*, 23, 336–343, 1980.

Rich, A., and Lerman, J., Teflon Laryngoplasty: An acoustical and perceptual study. *J. Speech Hearing Dis.*, 43, 496–505, 1978.

Riley, G., and Riley, J., Motoric and linguistic variables among children who stutter: a factor analysis. *J. Speech Hearing Dis.*, 45, 504–514, 1980.

Ruscello, D., and Shelton, R., Planning and self-assessment in articulatory training. *J. Speech Hearing Dis.*, 44, 504–512, 1979.

Schaeffer, M., and Shearer, W., A survey of mentally retarded stutterers. *Ment. Retardation*, 6, 44–45, 1968.

Schissel, R., and James, L. A comparison of children's performance on two tests of articulation. *J. Speech Hearing Dis.*, 44, 363–372, 1979.

Schmuach, V., Panagos, J., and Klick, R., Syntax influences the accuracy of consonant production in language-disordered children. *J. Communication Disorders*, 11, 315–323, 1978.

Schow, R., and Nerbonne, M., Hearing levels among elderly nursing home residents. *J. Speech Hearing Dis.*, 45, 124–132, 1980.

Senturia, B., and Wilson, F., Otorhinolaryngic findings in children with voice deviations. *Ann. Otol. Rhinol. Laryngol.*, 77, 1027–1042, 1968.

Shearer, W., Diagnosis and treatment of voice disorders in school children. *J. Speech Hearing Dis.*, 37, 215–221, 1972.

Shearer, W., and Simmons, B. Middle ear activity during speech in normal speakers and stutterers. *J. Speech Hearing Res.*, 8, 205–209, 1965.

Shearer, W., and Stevens, G., Acoustic threshold shift from power lawnmower noise. *Sound Vibration*, 3, 29, 1968.

Shearer, W., and Williams, D., Self-recovery from stuttering. *J. Speech Hearing Dis.*, 30, 288–290, 1965.

Sheehan, J., and Martyn, M., Stuttering and its disappearance. *J. Speech Hearing Res.*, 15, 297–298, 1970.

Shelton, R., Brooks, A., and Youngstrom, K. Clinical assessment of palatopharyngeal closure. *J. Speech Hearing Dis.*, 30, 37–43, 1965.

Shipp, T., Vertical laryngeal position during continuous and discrete vocal frequency change. *J. Speech Hearing Dis.*, 18, 707–718, 1975.

Siegel, G., Fehst, C., Garber, S., Pick, H., Delayed auditory feedback with children. *J. Speech Hearing Res.*, 23, 802–813, 1980.

Siegel, S., *Nonparametric Statistics for the Behavioral Sciences.* New York: McGraw-Hill, 1956.

Silverman, E., Listeners' impressions, of speakers with lateral lisps, *J. Speech Hearing Res.*, 41, 547–552, 1976.

Skinner, P., and Glottke, T., Electrophysiologic response audiometry: State of the art. *J. Speech Hearing Dis.*, 42, 179–198, 1977.

Sklar, M., Relation of psychological and language test scores and autopsy findings in aphasia. *J. Speech Hearing Dis.*, 6, 84–90, 1963.

Soderberg, G., Linguistics factors in stuttering. *J. Speech Hearing Res.*, 10, 801–810, 1967.

Soron, H., High-speed photography in speech research. *J. Speech Hearing Res.*, 10, 768–776, 1967.

Steele, R., and Torrie, J., *Principles and Procedures of Statistics*, New York: McGraw-Hill, 1960.

Stephens, I., Elicited imitation of selected features of two American English dialects in Head Start children. *J. Speech Hearing Res.*, 19, 493–508, 1976.

Stephens, I., and Daniloff, R., A methodological study of factors affecting the judgements of misarticulated /s/. *J. Communication Disorders*, 10, 207–220, 1977.

Stephen, S., and Haggard, M., Acoustic properties of masking/delayed feedback on the fluency of stutterers and controls. *J. Speech Hearing Res.*, 23, 527–538, 1980.

Studebaker, G., Clinical masking of air- and bone-conducted stimuli. *J. Speech Hearing Dis.*, 29, 23–35, 1964.

Studebaker, G., Clinical masking of the nontest ear. *J. Speech Hearing Dis.*, 32, 360–371, 1967.

Sweetow, R., and Barrager, D., Quality of comprehensive audiological care: a survey of hearing-impaired children. *ASHA*, 22, 841–848, 1980.

Townsend, T., Hearing aid measurements using the revised standard: Reducing variability and determining test system accuracy. *J. Speech Hearing Res.*, 23, 322–335, 1980.

Travis, L., *Speech Pathology*, New York: Appleton Co., 1931.

Trotter, W., and Silverman, F., The Stutterer as a character in contemporary literature: A bibliography. 1976.

Van Riper, C., *Speech Correction.* New York: Prentice-Hall, 1939.

Walden, b., Schuckman, G., and Sedge, R., The reliability and validity of the comfort level method of setting hearing aid gain. *J. Speech Hearing Dis.*, 42, 455–461, 1977.

Webster, R., and Lubker, B., Interrelationships among fluency producing variables in stuttered speech. *J. Speech Hearing Dis.*, 11, 754–766 (1968).

Weinberg, B., Shedd, D., and Harii, Y., Reed-fistula speech following pharyngolaryngectomy. *J. Speech Hearing Dis.*, 43, 401–413, 1978.

Weismer, G., and Longstreth, D., Segmental gestures at the laryngeal level of whispered speech. Evidence from an aerodynamic study. *J. Speech Hearing Res.*, 23, 383–392, 1980.

West, R., The *Rehabilitation of Speech.* New York: Harper Brothers, 1937.

Whitehead, R., and Barefoot, S., Some aerodynamic characteristics of plosive consonants produced by hearing-impaired speakers. *Amer. Ann. Deaf*, 125, 366–373, 1980.

Williams, D., personal communication, 1977.

Williams, J., Severity judgment of different types of simulated stuttering. Unpublished paper. Northern Illinois University, 1980.

Williams, J., and Martin, R., Immediate versus delayed consequences of stuttering responses. *J. Speech Hearing Res.*, 17, 569–575, 1974.

Winer, B., *Statistical Principles in Experimental Design.* New York: McGraw-Hill, 1962.

Winer, B., *Statistical Principles in Experimental Design.* (2nd Ed.,), New York: McGraw-Hill, 1971.

Wolf, K., and Goldstein, R., Middle component AERs from Neonates to low-level tonal stimuli. *J. Speech Hearing Res.*, 23, 185–201, 1980.

Wozniak, v., and Jackson, P., Visual vowel and diphthong perception from two horizontal viewing angles. *J. Speech Hearing Res.*, 22, 354–365, 1979.

Yates, J., Ramsey, J., and Holland, J. Damage Risk: An evaluation of the effects of exposure to 85 versus 90 dBA of voice. *J. Speech Hearing Res.*, 19, 216–224, 1976.

Young, M., Application of regression analysis concepts to retrospective research in speech pathology. *J. Speech Hearing Res.*, 19, 5–18, 1976.

Zurif, E., Lexical semantics and memory for words in aphasia. *J. Speech Hearing Res.*, 22, 465–467, 1979.

Author Index

Subject Index

DATE DUE

7 07 '83	
11 03 '83	

BRODART, INC.   Cat. No. 23-221